Real
YOGA

By
Vimla Lalvani

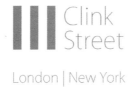

Clink Street

London | New York

Published by Clink Street Publishing 2016

Copyright © 2016

First edition.

ISBN: 978-1-911110-14-9
E-Book: 978-1-911110-15-6

Disclaimer

It is advisable to check with your doctor before embarking on any exercise program. Yoga should not be considered a replacement for professional medical treatment; a physician should be consulted in all matters relating to health and particularly in respect of pregnancy and any symptoms which may require diagnosis or medical attention. While the advice and information in this book are believed to be accurate and the step-by-step instructions have been devised to avoid strain, neither the author nor the publisher can accept any legal responsibility for any injury sustained while following the exercises.

For BKS Iyengar

Table of Contents

Prelude   6

Introduction   9

Breathing   18

Posture   21

Warm-Up   25

Relaxation   32

Course One   34
   Dog Pose   36
   The Tree   38
   The Eagle   39
   Standing Bow   40
   The Warrior   42
   Side Stretch   43
   Side Twist   44
   Flat Twist   45
   Leg Lifts   46
   The Fish   47
   Shoulder Stand   48
   The Cobra   50
   Cat Stretch   51
   The Camel   52
   The Rabbit   53
   Soles of the Feet   54
   Sitting Twist   55
   Pranayama   56

Course Two   58
   Head to Knee   60
   Knee Bends   62
   Side Leg Stretch   65
   Half-Moon   67
   Lunge with Balance   69
   Side Lunge   71
   The Tower   73
   Side Stretch   75
   Sitting Balance   78
   The Plough   80
   The Wheel   83
   Back Lift   84
   The Bow   85
   Spinal Twist   86
   Toe Pull   87
   Eye Exercise   88
   Total Stretch   89
   Uddiyana   91

Quick Fixes for Common Ailments   92
   Arthritis   94
   Osteoporosis   95
   Immune System   96
   Insomnia   97
   Depression   98
   Eye Strain   99
   Pelvic Floor   100
   Breaks & Fractures   101
   Thyroid   102
   Digestive   103

Spiritual Mindfulness   105
Visualisations & Meditations 107

Conclusion   113

Prelude

I was very privileged to meet as a child the greatest masters of wisdom. As my family was and still is the honorary consulates of India in Hawaii, I was introduced to Swami Mukhtanada, Swami, Chinmayadam, and a host of wsdom keepers that shared their knowledge with me. The Vedanta became a magical kingdom for me as my thirst of spiritual and philosophical knowledge grew.

Along with my passion for dance and movement, I longed to go to India to study Classical Indian dance under Master Kaliyanasudaram.

When I finished my studies, I traveled to Bombay to study Bharat Natyam. It was there that I experienced my first Yoga Class. Something inside me went click and I realized I found what I was looking for. The Connection made me feel whole. My mind, body, and spirit came together as one and I knew I could never turn back.

This was it! This is what I was looking for even without knowing it.

Yoga became my passion and my life's purpose. I gave up everything else and was determined to find the greatest Living Master to train me.

Unbelievably, he was on my doorstep.

As I don't believe in coincidences I knew that this was to become my life's path.

My Master, BKS Iyengar, was a huge challenge for me. In those days there was no such thing as paying for tuition. The Master had to offer you his tutelage and there was nothing you could do to persuade or convince him.

I tried so hard. I went every day to his classroom and was turned down, thrown out, and on many occasions shouted at to leave to never return.

I cried and pleaded and it was always no. However, I never gave up.

One day, I decided to disguise myself as an Indian with kurta pajamas and braided hair. I look back at the incident and recall how silly I behaved as I am Indian and how would he not recognize that I was the same girl from Hawaii in an Indian outfit.

I think he was amused as he did not comment on my existence or me as the class began.

I was in a perfect shoulder stand when Iyengar pulled me up from the floor and swung me around like a cat. I told you to get out he retorted. I was terrified and froze in fear. He placed me done gently

6

and I nearly broke out in tears.

The other students pleaded with him. Let her stay. She is so young and she is good!

That was it. He let me stay and he trained me with precise discipline which his method is known for. The first time I saw him in the distance, without knowing that it was the Master himself, Iyengar exuded such powerful energy force that would bowl you over. His charisma was so dynamic and there was a shine around his face.

Even though he was strict and fearsome, I will be ever grateful to him for his personal training and wisdom. I know now that he wanted to challenge me. To make sure he was not wasting time on someone who would not make it his or her life's path.

When I completed my training, after one year, he said now you go home and teach.

I said Masterji, who will listen to me. I am so young (20 years old)

He replied. Don't worry child, the whole world will listen. And here I still am and yes, the world did listen.

After the writing of my many books and producing my DVD's. Iyengar was on a trip to London and asked the head of the Iyengar School in London to go out and purchase every single Yoga product that I have produced.

She called me to say that Iyengar had asked to see, read, and watch every single book, video, and DVD that I had ever produced. I always acknowledged him on every product but this was the real test: His approval.

I was shaking throughout the afternoon not knowing the outcome.

She eventually called and said Congratulations. Masterji has asked me to thank you for all the good work you have done to bring Yoga to the World. Please tell her that what she has done I could not do as she has brought Yoga to the masses with her modern vision.

I collapsed in tears. What a relief. Was it pride? Was it approval I was seeking? I felt like that young girl again.

But this was different. This was from thankfulness to God to give me such an opportunity in life. To give me purpose in life from which I have never waivered.

Thank you my dear Masterji for believing in me and giving me your knowledge and wisdom to teach Yoga to the World.

Every human being has a divine spark. My job is to ignite this deep glow with divine Light.

Vimla

INTRODUCTION

Introduction

WHAT IS YOGA?

Many people want to know what yoga is and how it can help them. In this book I hope to explain classical yoga in a modern sense and to de-mystify the principles of yoga philosophy. The benefits of yoga are many and people who practice regularly will see a great change in their physical body and their whole mental outlook.

Given the stresses and strains of our daily lives, we must learn the art of shutting ourselves away from chaos and retreating into our inner selves to find peace, balance and harmony. Yoga teaches you how to achieve this. Classic Yoga explains how yoga can improve your everyday life. You will discover the real you and experience 'yoga living'. You will learn the techniques of yoga and understand the mental and physical aspects of the philosophy.

In Sanskrit, the word 'yoga' means the union of mind and body. Yoga is not a religion but a philosophy of life. It is an ancient science of movement developed in India thousands of years ago to improve all aspects of your life, both mental and physical. The main principle of yoga is that mastery over the mind and senses will lead to a cessation of misery and bring you salvation.

THE PATHS OF YOGA

There are five different forms of yoga and for maximum benefit they should be practiced together. The four mental yogas are Bhakti yoga (emotions), Gyana yoga (wisdom), Raja yoga (meditation) and Karma yoga (actions). The one physical yoga is called Hatha yoga. In this book we concentrate on Hatha yoga because it is the first stage of development; yoga philosophy states that before you can have a disciplined mind you must first begin to train your body.

Hatha yoga is a series of asanas, or postures, that train and discipline the body and mind. In Sanskrit, 'ha' means the sun or male energy and 'tha' the moon or female energy. When you practice the asanas you are combining and balancing the masculine and feminine energies which are within all of us, whether male or female. In the Western world today, where professions, tasks and hobbies that were once considered exclusively

'masculine' or 'feminine' are largely shared by men and women, it is essential that both energies are balanced equally. Yoga is the art and science of balance in everyday living and moderation in all that we do. It teaches us how to have harmonious relationships with others and how to understand our own inner truth. It connects us to our souls and sets us on a path of true spirituality. The ultimate goal for the yogi is to join the spiritual self to the cosmic energy of the universe.

HATHA YOGA

Hatha yoga exercises the glands, organs and nerves in the body as well as toning the muscles. The yoga exercises are divided between asanas (exercise positions), Pranayama (breath control), Raj asanas (meditative postures), and Nauli, Mudras and Bandhas (purifying and cleansing postures). The exercises might appear strange when you first begin but as you familiarize yourself with the sequences you will understand how they work. Fluid movements unblock energy and, combined with correct breathing, increase your vitality and discipline your mind.

YOGA FOR TODAY

The popularity of yoga has soared in recent years. Attitudes to health, spirituality, lifestyle and mankind's place in the environment have changed dramatically and people are seeking solutions to the problems of their everyday existence. In these confusing times, the environment is struggling for survival and we are suffering from mental and physical stress, with some new diseases making an appearance and old ones thought to have been conquered by antibiotics reasserting themselves. We cannot always change these conditions but we can learn to cope with them. Yoga provides a perfect solution because it brings harmony and balance to your life; because your mental state is balanced you will be able to solve problems calmly and rationally, and because your physical health is improved you will have a better resistance to illnesses.

The yoga system is based on universal truths, so it does not interfere with anyone's religious beliefs. Yoga is for men and women of all ages and occupations and you can begin to learn at any time. Everyone's life is transformed and enriched by a new outlook, improved health, a new awareness and a fresh philosophy.

THE PHYSICAL BENEFITS OF YOGA

Yoga is totally different from other types of exercise. First of all, it is non-competitive. The purpose of yoga is to understand yourself through your yoga practice and to work slowly and deliberately to gain flexibility as you progress. It is the antithesis of the 'no pain, no gain' philosophy. Graceful, fluid movements replace pounding flesh, creating a balance and strength of the mind, body and spirit.

The purpose is not to build muscle but to build muscle tone. In yoga asanas the muscles are stretched lengthwise. Fat is eliminated around the cells and, combined with correct breathing, the exercises will improve the circulation and release toxin build-up. This process will reduce cellulite.

Yoga asanas also regulate the metabolism which controls weight gain and loss. As we grow older the metabolism slows down automatically. Continued practice of yoga postures keeps the metabolism rate stable so your weight will not fluctuate, and you will be able to maintain your ideal weight. Yoga also builds the immune system, so you will rarely experience even a common cold, and exercises the internal organs so that the body will work like a finely tuned car which runs in peak condition.

Yoga also helps to ease physical tensions through deep stretching and correct breathing techniques. Working on the physical body with deep concentration on breathing creates a real and lasting sense of harmony, embracing the body and mind. Yoga is a wonderful way of learning how to relax.

The physical techniques create a calm and concentration that extend beyond the body deep into the mind, effectively reducing stress at all levels.

DIET AND LIFESTYLE

Many people believe that in order to begin studying yoga they must change their habits. They may well fear that they will be told to give up meat, alcohol and smoking overnight! In fact, yoga is not about abstinence at all – rather, it is about the art of moderation.

In yoga, there are no fixed rules laid down about what is permissible. However, because the philosophy is about returning your body to its natural equilibrium you will not feel the need for excesses. When your mind and body are in harmony and you are in tune with yourself you will want to maintain a healthy, balanced lifestyle.

Many people are quite content to continue with Hatha yoga and benefit from the new-found discipline. Others discover a need to go further. Yoga opens the mind to a certain stillness and clarity and many people find they wish to pursue a spiritual path. Yoga raises the conscious level and brings the soul, mind and body into union by means of eight disciplines: Yama (ethics); Niyama (religious observances); Asana (postures); Pranayama (breathing

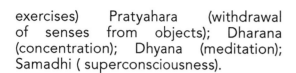

exercises) Pratyahara (withdrawal of senses from objects); Dharana (concentration); Dhyana (meditation); Samadhi (superconsciousness).

THE CHAKRAS

In the Sanskrit language, the word 'chakra' means 'wheel'. Chakras are 'wheels' that radiate energy in a circular motion through the vital centres of the spine. Just as antennae are able to pick up radio waves and transform them into sound, so chakras pick up cosmic vibrations and distribute them throughout the body via these energy centers.

In the spine we have seven chakras or energy centers moving from the tail bone up to the top of the head. Each center controls different senses, and all these centers must flow freely to maintain good health.

Many people have blocked chakras, and yoga exercises unblock them. The twisting and turning of the body stretches the nerves and the increased supply of oxygen cleanses and purifies the bloodstream. Every cell is renewed and the energy flows smoothly.

I like to use a hosepipe as an analogy. When there is a kink in the pipe the water will trickle out slowly and unevenly; when the pipe is unkinked the water will flow strongly. It is exactly the same in the case of energy. When the chakras are unblocked the energy flow will be powerful and dynamic.

It is important for you to be able to visualize the energy moving through your spine and there is a technique that will allow you to experience this. Sit upright on the floor, preferably in a cross-legged or lotus position. Look over your surroundings, close your eyes and relax the muscles of your face. Begin to breathe deeply and slowly. Become aware of the energy in the base of your spine. Feel bliss, calm and serenity. Stretch your arms out to the sides of your body with your palms facing upward. Gradually raise your arms and visualize the energy slowly moving to the center of your spine, then between the shoulder blades, up through the base of your neck and on through to the very top of your head. Clasp your hands over your head and continue to stretch your arms up while keeping your knees and shoulders down. Feel your fingertips tingling with energy and release your hands in a sudden burst. You will be surprised at how energized and powerful you feel as a result of carrying out this simple exercise.

All yogic exercises are based on a formula of stretching, relaxation and deep breathing to increase the circulation and improve concentration. In the meditative poses, sitting while breathing deeply reduces the metabolic rate. When the body is kept in this steady pose for some time, the mind becomes free of physiological disturbances caused by physical activity. There is a steady flow of nerve energy that electrifies the body and awakens the spiritual power in man through breathing techniques and concentration. The Raj asanas prepare you for meditation – focusing your mind on one thought. It is a scientific approach that you can apply to many areas of your life. When you rid your mind of useless thoughts, clarity is increased and you can find your own solutions rather than relying on a third party. This is one of the goals of the aspiring yogi. You will experience the power and joy of yoga when you can master your own thoughts and actions.

HOW TO USE THIS BOOK

For this book I have specifically designed two Yoga courses, which are based on different levels of fitness and experience of yoga. Before you begin Course One, it is important that you familiarize with the safety guidelines (page ?), breath control (page?) and correct posture (page?) Before embarking on any course you should follow the warm-up page (page ?) and cool down afterwards with a relaxation routine (page ?)

Course One is a foundation course in which you will learn the importance of breathing correctly and of aligning the spine. The yoga exercises are very gentle, slow and easy to follow, and will teach you to move in a new way. These exercises are linked to a specific breathing pattern, which will allow your energy to alter and flow freely through the system. Keep your mind focused on what your body is doing to create the link between mental and physical. Even though these exercises will be new, always keep your mind calm and pay attention to how you feel while you are doing each exercise. You will know immediately what mental state you are in- some days you will be surprised by your skill and other days you might need a sense of humor! As you are different every day, so your yoga practice will be too; the most important aspect to bear in mind is never become discouraged. Each day is a new day and as you become familiar with the sequences, your yoga practice will strengthen and deepen.

When you are sure you have thoroughly mastered Course One you can move on to Course Two. This Course presents you with more dynamic exercises, which, you will easily discover, call for more strength, stamina, and suppleness. As you move into the more challenging yoga asanas, you will feel a sense of elation in your ability to tackle these difficult poses; you will become energized and motivated, yet your mood will be calm.

You will probably find that not only

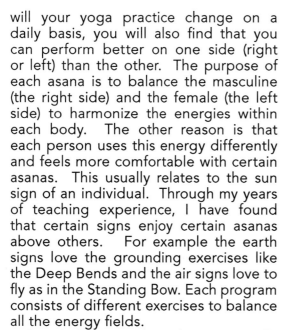

will your yoga practice change on a daily basis, you will also find that you can perform better on one side (right or left) than the other. The purpose of each asana is to balance the masculine (the right side) and the female (the left side) to harmonize the energies within each body. The other reason is that each person uses this energy differently and feels more comfortable with certain asanas. This usually relates to the sun sign of an individual. Through my years of teaching experience, I have found that certain signs enjoy certain asanas above others. For example the earth signs love the grounding exercises like the Deep Bends and the air signs love to fly as in the Standing Bow. Each program consists of different exercises to balance all the energy fields.

The rule here is to do each asana equally well regardless whether you like it or not. Pay attention to the one's you find difficult and challenging as these are the one's you need the most to rebalance. Yoga is a discipline, so only continued practice will show results.

These results will be dynamic; an invigorated body, increased stamina, improved muscle tone and a feeling of total harmony and calm.

There is another branch of Yoga called remedial Yoga in which doctors and chiropractors prescribe certain exercises to alleviate pain from chronic conditions.

I have taken some of the most common ailments and have suggested a certain exercise to first relieve the pain and second to use as a preventive measure from further attacks. Yoga is a preventive science to keep the body fit and healthy.

Daily practice will strengthen the immune system. Yoga improves blood supply to the internal organs rejuvenating all the cells. Combined with a healthy organic diet, this is the best you can do for yourself to prevent disease and illness.

Mindfulness is a buzzword today, but has been practiced for thousands of years.

I am including simple ways to train the mind to focus and concentrate. It is normal to have a thousand thoughts circling through the mind and it takes discipline to learn how to concentrate on one thought: that is the art of meditation. It is a brilliant tool and anyone can learn to do this. The Yoga method includes breath control and candle gazing.

Yoga practice eventually leads to a spiritual path and I have included some visualization exercises to encourage you to experience bliss. When you learn to connect to the divine, a new world opens up to you. With new eyes, you experience I am the Presence. There is divine wisdom in each and every one of us. This intelligence draws us to the Light. Yoga awakens the Infinite Wisdom Within to shift our perception of life. Love exudes from our hearts to see everything and everyone as One. There is no separation of thoughts, as no imperfections or darkness can exist when the Body of Light shines from your soul. Light is Life. Oneness is Light.

Make it your Calling to seek this wisdom that is available to us all. It is your Divine right to experience the serenity of inner tranquility and Yoga brings to you the tools to make this possible.

EXPLANATION OF TERMS

- For first position, stand tall in perfect posture with your feet together.
- For second position, stand tall in perfect posture with your feet apart, directly under the hip bones, and toes pointing forward. If an exercise calls for wide second position, place your feet 1–1.2m (3–4ft) apart.
- To center yourself, concentrate on the solar plexus while breathing deeply. This helps to balance your physical and mental state.
- To lift your spine, concentrate on the tail bone (the coccyx) while lifting your spine straight.
- To open the chest, push your shoulder blades down and lift the chest naturally to create a positive outlook.
- If an exercise calls for a flat back, your spine should be straight and parallel to the floor.

- Lotus position: the classic posture for meditation and pranayama. Sitting with your spine erect, bend your knees and cross your ankles in front of you.
- For the half lotus, pull one foot up high onto the opposite thigh and place the second foot under the thigh of your first leg.
- For the full lotus, place the second leg over the first, with the foot high on the opposite thigh and your knees touching the floor.
- The half lotus can also be assumed in a standing position and the full lotus can be performed sitting, or in the head and shoulder stands.

SAFETY GUIDELINES

Here are some important guidelines which must always be followed in order to make sure that you are able to gain all the benefits that yoga has to offer and do not inadvertently injure yourself by exercising incorrectly.

- The yoga courses in this book have been designed for people who are in a normal state of health. As is the case with any fitness program, if you feel unfit or unwell or you are recovering from an illness or injury, are pregnant, have high blood pressure or suffer from any medical disorder you must consult your doctor before embarking upon any of the exercises.

- Always follow the course exactly and do the exercises in the right order, and always begin your practice with the warm-up to help loosen the muscles. Exercising stiff muscles leads to injury.
- Never rush the movements and follow the directions exactly. Do not jerk your body and stop immediately if you experience any sharp pain or strain to any muscle.
- Never push yourself and always do the pose only to your own capability. Remember that yoga is strictly non-competitive and, if you are following these courses with a friend, don't succumb to the temptation to go at the same rate of progress as him or her if it doesn't suit you. It is for you to find your own pace.
- Pay particular attention to your breathing in order to help relax and focus your mind. Pay special attention to your posture, too, and make sure that you always stand, sit or kneel upright.
- When you are carrying out a standing exercise you will often be required to balance upon one leg. Keep the leg on which you are standing straight by lifting the muscle above the kneecap. Do not hyper-extend the knee because this can cause injury.
- Do not exercise on a full stomach.

You must wait four hours after a heavy meal or one hour after a light snack.

- Choose a warm, quiet, well-ventilated place in which to exercise. Wear clothing that you can comfortably stretch in. All yoga exercises are done in bare feet so that you can grip the floor with your toes. You might need a mat for the floor work, but otherwise just make sure you exercise on an even, non-slip surface.
- After exercising, the body always needs a cooling down period to return it to normal. Always finish with the relaxation pose, even if just for a short time. However, the longer the relaxation period you can manage the better as deep breathing restores the equilibrium and calms the nervous system.
- Whenever you practice yoga, remember these basic principles: soul/mind control of movements; awareness of postures and movements; slow and deliberate movements; relaxation during movements; positive non-competitive attitude; go only as far as is comfortable.

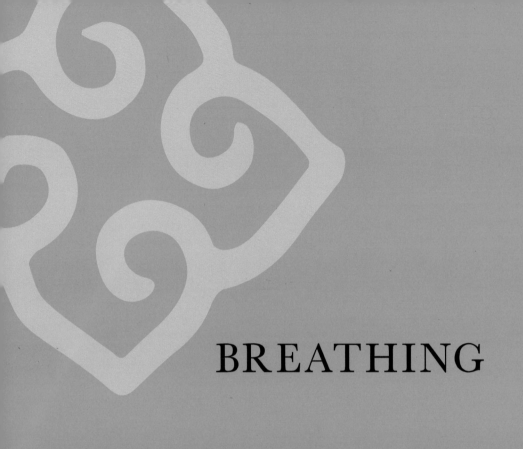

BREATHING

Breathing

Learning the art of correct breathing is vital to your health and well-being. In yoga we breathe from the diaphragm. If you watch a baby breathe you can see the diaphragm rise and fall, but adults tend to breathe from the chest. When you breathe correctly you increase lung capacity and send more oxygen into the bloodstream, revitalizing and purifying the internal organs. Correct breathing acts as a natural tranquillizer to the nervous system; the deeper you breathe the calmer your mind becomes. Keep the breath even and always breathe through the nose, never the mouth unless specifically instructed.

1

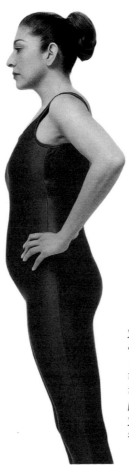

Stand in perfect posture. Inhale deeply and push your stomach out from the diaphragm. Do not move your chest, and keep your shoulders down.

2

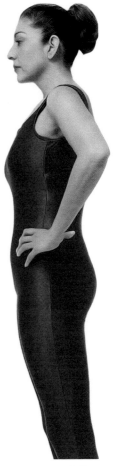

Exhale deeply. Keep your breathing steady and even. Repeat Steps 1 and 2 for at least 10 full breaths. Always follow this breathing pattern before you start your yoga practice, to steady your mind.

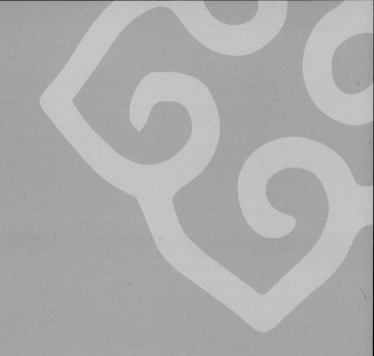

POSTURE

Posture

One of the basics of yoga is to sit and stand in perfect posture, and many poses are designed to strengthen the muscles in the lower back so that you are able to lift your spine in perfect alignment. Whether you are sitting, standing or kneeling, think of a string pulling you up from the crown of your head. Always 'open the chest' by pushing your shoulder blades down, lifting the chest naturally. The basic standing pose is called Tadasana, which means 'the mountain'. It is a dynamic pose and you should be aware of every muscle in the body. Stand with your feet together and your weight evenly distributed between your toes and heels. Pull your stomach in, tuck your buttocks under and lift the muscle above the kneecaps. Keep your arms at your sides, elbows straight and fingertips together. To test yourself, balance on your toes; you should not fall backward or forward.

1

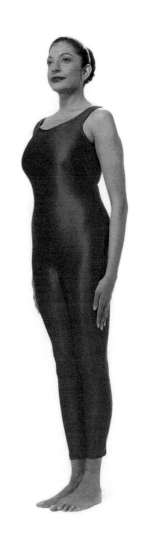

Stand in perfect posture. Inhale deeply and push your stomach out from the diaphragm. Do not move your chest, and keep your shoulders down.

2

Exhale deeply. Keep your breathing steady and even. Repeat Steps 1 and 2 for at least 10 full breaths. Always follow this breathing pattern before you start your yoga practice, to steady your mind.

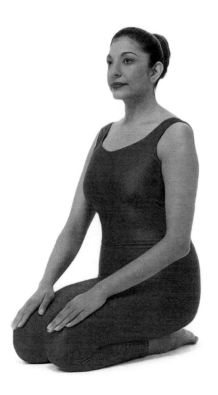

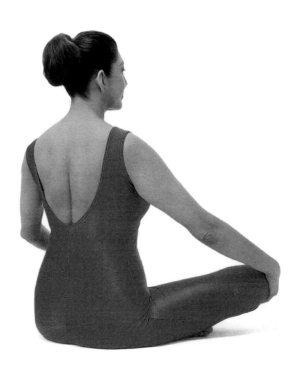

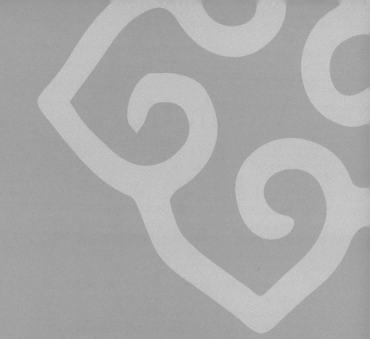

WARM-UP

Warm-Up

It is always essential to warm up the body slowly and gently before beginning the yoga course of your choice. This series of movements combined with breathing in the correct manner will help to loosen the spine and gently prepare your body for the other exercises that follow. Before you begin, focus attention on yourself and breathe deeply from your diaphragm for ten seconds. 'Center' – that is, focus on balancing your physical and mental state – by assuming a good posture. You need to stand evenly with your weight balanced between your toes and heels.

As you do the exercises you will feel the energy flow freely from one movement to the next.

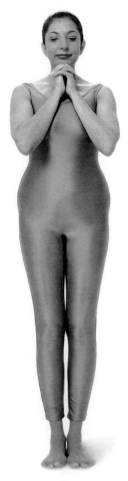

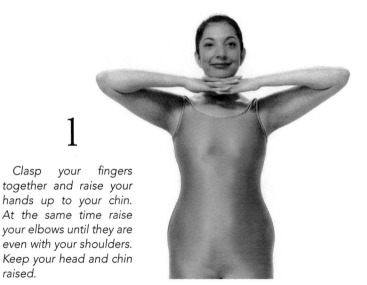

1

Clasp your fingers together and raise your hands up to your chin. At the same time raise your elbows until they are even with your shoulders. Keep your head and chin raised.

2

Inhale and breathe deeply, bringing your elbows down toward each other. Make sure you don't drop your chin. Exhale and return to Step 1.

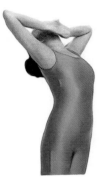

3

Drop your head back, raise your elbows and clasp your hands under your chin.

4

Inhale and breathe deeply, bringing the elbows together. Exhale and return to Step 3.

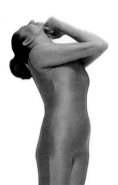

5

Bring your clasped hands down, inhale and then raise your arms above your head and exhale.

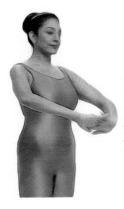

6

Keep your chin up and shoulders down as you stretch your spine fully by reaching your arms as high as possible. Slowly inhale and exhale.

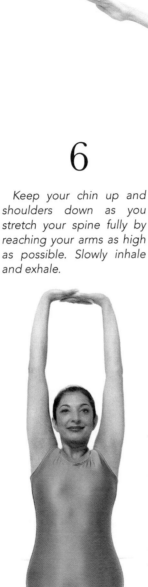

7

Put your arms down by your sides, then inhale and stretch your left arm over to the right, keeping the hips square. Exhale and stretch downward, extending the right hand toward the floor. Continue inhaling and exhaling and stretch in both directions for 5 seconds. Then repeat on the other side.

8

Put your arms behind your back and hold firmly onto your elbows with your opposite hand. Slowly inhale and exhale.

9

Inhale, push your hips forward and drop your head back, transferring your weight toward your heels. Keep your toes on the ground.

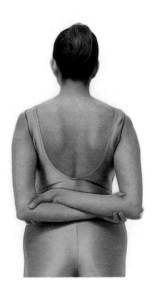

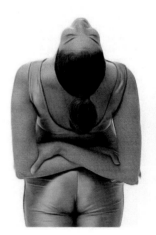

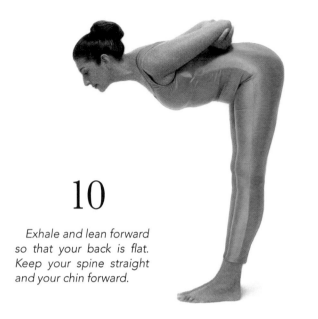

10

Exhale and lean forward so that your back is flat. Keep your spine straight and your chin forward.

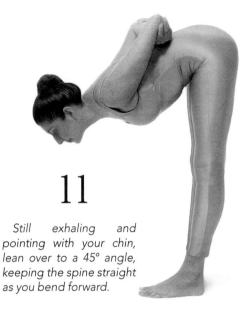

11

Still exhaling and pointing with your chin, lean over to a 45° angle, keeping the spine straight as you bend forward.

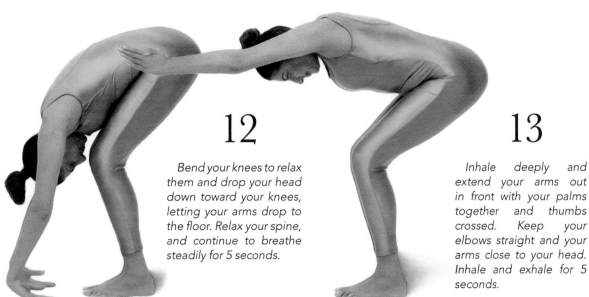

12

Bend your knees to relax them and drop your head down toward your knees, letting your arms drop to the floor. Relax your spine, and continue to breathe steadily for 5 seconds.

13

Inhale deeply and extend your arms out in front with your palms together and thumbs crossed. Keep your elbows straight and your arms close to your head. Inhale and exhale for 5 seconds.

14

Return to a standing position, lift your arms high over your head and clasp your palms together.

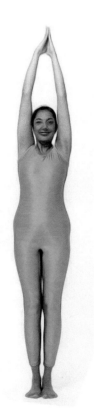

15

Inhale and as you exhale stretch all the way over to the right side. Keep your head evenly balanced between your arms and your feet together on the ground. Hold for 5 seconds, breathing normally. Inhale and return to Step 14. Repeat on the other side.

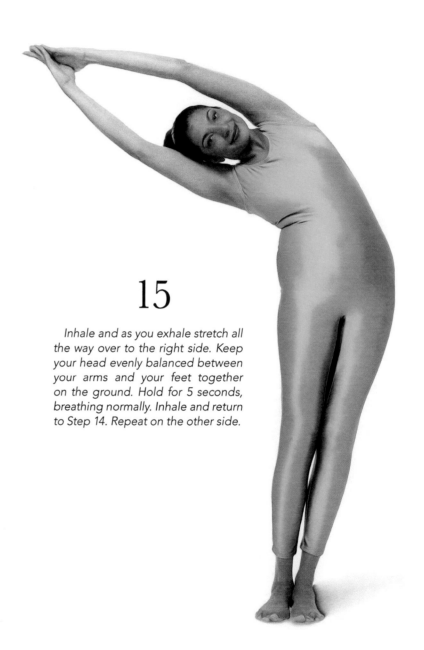

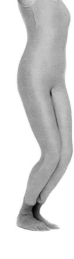

17

Return to the Step 14 position and keep your arms above your head. Now bend your knees, while breathing steadily.

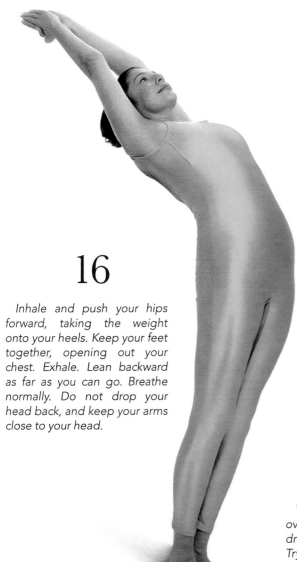

16

Inhale and push your hips forward, taking the weight onto your heels. Keep your feet together, opening out your chest. Exhale. Lean backward as far as you can go. Breathe normally. Do not drop your head back, and keep your arms close to your head.

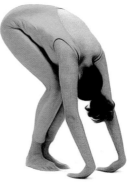

18

With knees bent, lean over to relax your body, dropping your arms down. Try to put your forehead on your knees. Uncurl and relax.

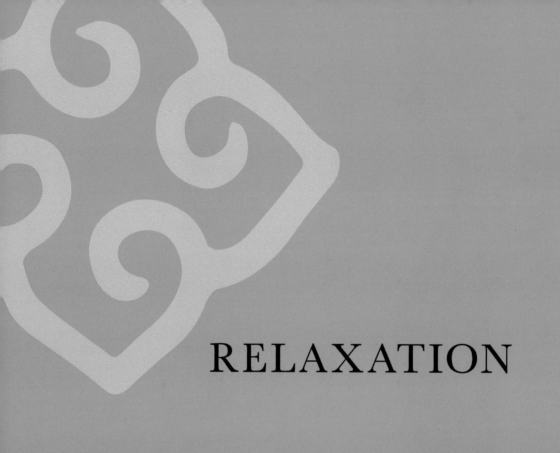

RELAXATION

Relaxation

Learning the art of relaxation is essential to your well-being. These techniques not only help to rejuvenate the body but also release stress and tension in the muscle groups and calm the nerves. If you use the breathing exercise in the middle of the day it will refresh your mind and body. If you do it at night before you go to sleep, it can help cure insomnia. To release stress and tension in the muscle groups, begin by first focusing on your diaphragm and breathe deeply and slowly for 15 seconds. On every exhalation you'll feel the tension release from your body. Concentrate your mind on a pleasant image, such as a beautiful beach. Now concentrate on your feet and tense and release your toes. Flex your feet hard and as you relax them you'll feel the tension release in your ankles, knees, thighs, buttocks and stomach muscles. Repeat with your hands, tightening the arms and elbows while gripping your hands in a tight fist. Now raise your shoulder blades up and then relax them down again. Repeat twice. Next turn your head slowly to the right and slowly to the left, then let your head flop down. Finally, relax the face muscles, breathing deeply and keeping calm.

1

This is the dead man's pose. Lie flat on the floor with the palms of your hands facing upward and make sure your feet and legs are relaxed. Stay in this position for 15 minutes for the maximum benefit.

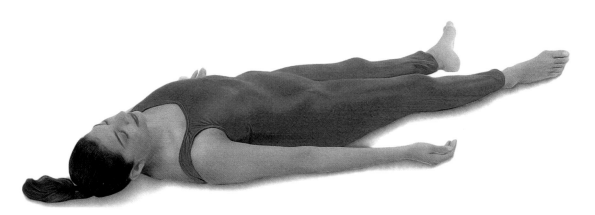

COURSE
ONE

Course One

INTRODUCTION

Course One is a foundation course for total beginners. It will teach you to balance your mental and physical energies and increase your flexibility and muscle tone, while improving your body shape and relaxing your nervous system.

Yoga is a science of movement: you should always begin with the Warm-up (see above), and the exercises must be followed in their exact order. In Course 1 you are introduced slowly to the system with easy poses and stretches which will familiarize you with the yoga way of movement; you should pay special attention to details like hand and feet positions.

Remember that even when you do not feel as if you are moving, yoga is never static. Modern physical exercises like aerobics require a lot of energy, as every violent move burns it up; lactic acids are formed in the muscle fibers and this tires the muscles. The slow movements of yoga waste no energy; deep breathing allows more oxygen absorption and muscles suffer no fatigue.

Concentrate on what your body is doing. This is the first step toward disciplining the mind and body.

Dog Pose

This exercise is wonderful for stretching the whole body. Not only does it increase blood circulation, it also helps to tone and strengthen the legs and arms as well as curing fatigue and increasing your vitality. As with all the downward poses, it calms the nervous system and can be used as a relaxation pose if you're tired. Breathe deeply and evenly throughout the movements and relax your neck to release any tension in the shoulders.

1

Sit back on your heels with your toes curled under. Stretch out your arms in front of you and straighten your elbows. Place your forehead on the floor.

2

Inhale and kneel up, keeping your hands balanced out in front of you. Exhale and breathe normally. Stretch your fingers evenly on the floor, and keep your knees under the hips.

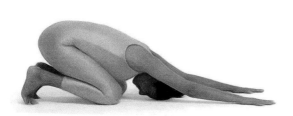

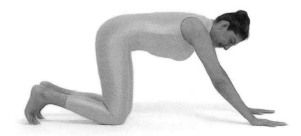

4

Now flatten your heels on the floor and move your thighs outward. Lift up your knees and stretch your spine upward. Straighten your arms and keep your shoulders down. Relax your face and neck, and breathe deeply for 30–60 seconds. As you gain flexibility, hold for longer. Relax and slowly stand upright.

3

Inhale, push the palms down and raise your hips upward. Stretch high onto your toes, pushing the shoulder blades down. Open out the chest and release the neck and shoulders. Bring your head in line with your spine and push your hips back. Hold for 10 seconds, while breathing normally.

The Tree

This standing pose focuses your mind and helps you learn how to concentrate and balance steadily on one leg. By balancing properly, you challenge your mind and you can unite your mental and physical energies. It also teaches you the importance of distributing your weight evenly between your heels and toes.

2

Look straight ahead and try to balance comfortably. When you are absolutely still, place your palms together and hold for 5 seconds. Grip the floor firmly with your toes so that the ankle does not move from side to side.

1

Stand up straight. Place your right foot on your inner left thigh or close to the ankle or knee. Push out your hip but keep your hips square. Place your left hand on your left hip. Lift your standing leg as high as possible by stretching the muscle above the kneecap.

3

Now stretch your arms right up, while holding your balance for 5 seconds. Feel the energy move from your heels through your legs, into the spine and then through your arms and fingertips. Repeat on the other side.

The Eagle

The Eagle exercise focuses your mind so that you can concentrate on attention to detail. It grounds your energy and improves your balance. It can help to eliminate any cellulite and extra fat around the thighs, and also tones the leg, arm, and calf muscles. As you do the exercise, always keep your eyes fixed ahead on one spot to help you maintain your balance.

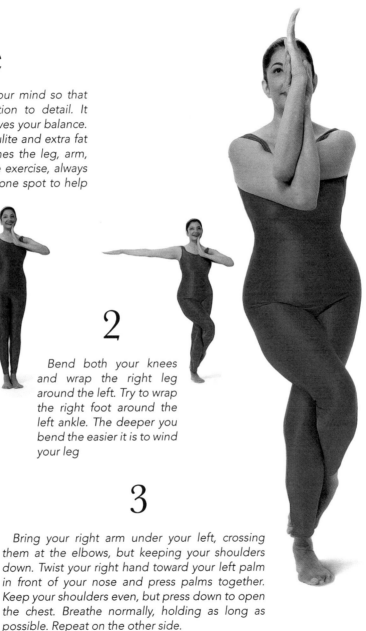

1

Stand up straight. Hold your left hand, facing upward, in front of your nose and stretch out your right arm. Focus on one spot straight ahead. Breathe normally.

2

Bend both your knees and wrap the right leg around the left. Try to wrap the right foot around the left ankle. The deeper you bend the easier it is to wind your leg

3

Bring your right arm under your left, crossing them at the elbows, but keeping your shoulders down. Twist your right hand toward your left palm in front of your nose and press palms together. Keep your shoulders even, but press down to open the chest. Breathe normally, holding as long as possible. Repeat on the other side.

Standing Bow

This graceful exercise, called the Standing Bow because of the curve of the spine, will give you a sense of elation and power when you hold the pose as long as possible. The energy is continuously flowing in a circular pattern and as you increase the stretch your breathing pattern will quicken. Breathe deeply from the diaphragm to increase energy levels. This exercise will rejuvenate your spine and give you a sense of joy. Your circulation will be greatly improved and your whole body toned.

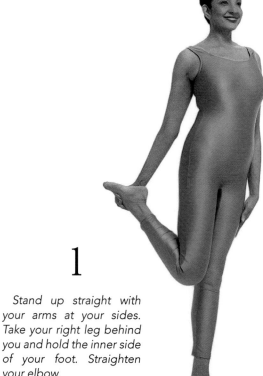

1

Stand up straight with your arms at your sides. Take your right leg behind you and hold the inner side of your foot. Straighten your elbow.

2

Take your left arm up close to your ear. Keep both shoulders down and look straight ahead. Breathe normally and steady your balance.

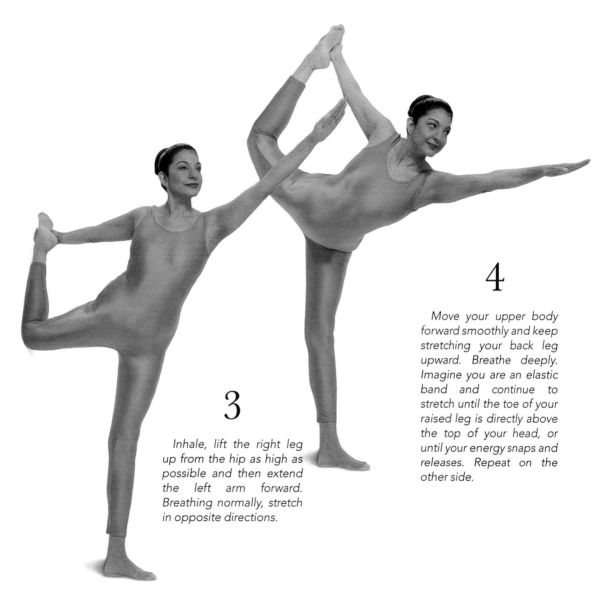

4

Move your upper body forward smoothly and keep stretching your back leg upward. Breathe deeply. Imagine you are an elastic band and continue to stretch until the toe of your raised leg is directly above the top of your head, or until your energy snaps and releases. Repeat on the other side.

3

Inhale, lift the right leg up from the hip as high as possible and then extend the left arm forward. Breathing normally, stretch in opposite directions.

41

The Warrior

The Warrior pose is dynamic in its approach, and its aim is to develop a positive mental attitude and to give you physical control over your body. The Warrior is the basis for all standing postures, so the exact positioning of your spine, arms, legs and feet is very important. Hold your spine very straight as you open out your chest.

1

Stand up straight, feet together, and bend your knees slightly in preparation to jump. Bring your arms up to shoulder level and place your fingertips together.

2

Jump to open your legs wide – they should be about 1.2m (4ft) apart. Make sure your toes are pointing forward and stretch both your arms out sideways.

3

Turn your right knee and foot to the right. Lean your body backward and push your hips and stomach forward. Now bend your right knee, keeping your spine straight. Bend further until there is a 90° angle between your thigh and the floor. Repeat on the other side.

Side Stretch

Stretching to the side is an exercise that improves every muscle, joint, tendon and organ in the body. It also revitalizes the nerves, veins and body tissue by increasing the flow of oxygen to the blood. It helps cure sciatica, lumbago and other lower-back ailments. The body's strength and flexibility is heightened by the deep stretching, especially in the hip joints, waist and torso.

1

Stand up straight and place your feet about 1m (3ft) apart. Stretch out your arms with your palms facing down. Keep them in line with your shoulders. Breathe normally.

2

Turn in your left foot slightly and point your right foot 90° to the right. Inhale and stretch to the right. Keep the spine straight and do not tilt forward. Breathe normally and hold for 5 seconds.

3

Place your right hand on your right ankle and extend your left arm up in a straight line with your palm facing forward. Look up toward your arm, keeping your head up. Relax your face and shoulders, and hold for 10 seconds

Side Twist

The standing twist helps to tone the leg muscles and waist, as well as relieving back pain and other ailments such as sciatica and lumbago.

The twisting motion invigorates the abdominal organs and releases any toxins from the system. Remember to keep both legs straight as you twist from the hip upward.

1

Stand upright with your feet about 1.2m (4ft) apart and your toes pointing forward. Hold your arms out level with your shoulders and stretch out as far as you can.

2

Now turn sideways to the left, pointing out your left foot. Make sure your heel is in line with the right foot's instep. Still keep your arms outstretched.

3

Now hold your left ankle with your right hand and look over your left shoulder. Keep your arms in a straight line. Hold for 10 seconds and then repeat on the other side. Breathe normally throughout.

Flat Twist

The Flat Twist relieves any tension that gets trapped in the neck and shoulders. It also alleviates lower back pain and is a really good stretching exercise for your spine. Remember to keep both shoulders flat on the ground and always look in the opposite direction to your feet to increase the body stretch.

1

Lie flat on the ground and take your arms out to the side, placing your palms facing down. Put your left heel on top of the toes of the right foot. Breathe normally.

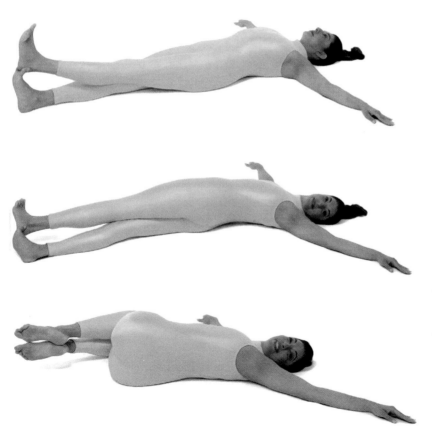

2

Inhale and as you exhale twist both feet to the right and look over your left shoulder. Hold the position for 5 seconds.

3

Bend your knees into your chest to increase the stretch, keeping legs and feet together. Inhale as your legs come up and then exhale and twist to the left. Relax onto your back and repeat on the other side.

Leg Lifts

These exercises will tone your stomach and leg muscles and improve the flexibility of your hamstrings and spine. It might be quite difficult in the beginning to achieve Step 3, but with continued practice you will be able to release all the stiffness in your joints.

2

Put your hands around your ankle, if you can, and stretch further, trying to place your forehead on your knee. Trying to keep both legs straight and breathing normally, hold for 10 seconds. Repeat Steps 1 and 2 on the other side.

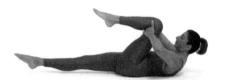

1

Lie on the floor. Clasp your hands behind your left knee and bring it into your chest. Lift your head up from the floor toward the knee. Point your toes and lift your right leg just off the floor. Breathe normally and hold for 5 seconds.

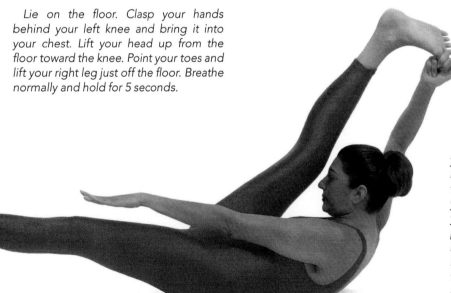

3

Clasp your fingers around your big toe and pull your right leg even further toward your head, keeping your right foot flexed. Take your left arm out, with your palm facing down, and hold just above your left leg. Breathe deeply, hold for 10 seconds and repeat on the other side.

The Fish

When you do the Fish exercise you'll tone the stomach and leg muscles as well as releasing tension in the neck and shoulders. It also improves circulation to the face and slows the ageing process. These movements strengthen the lower back and open out the chest, increasing your lung capacity, which improves conditions such as bronchitis and asthma.

1

Lie on the floor with your arms out and point your toes. Inhale and raise your chest, resting your weight on the crown of your head. Feel the stretch in your neck and face. Exhale and breathe normally, holding for 3 seconds.

2

Still balancing on your head, inhale and raise your right leg, keeping your hip on the floor. Place your palms together above your chest, holding for 3 seconds. As you exhale, lower your leg slowly. Relax to the floor, if necessary, before Step 3.

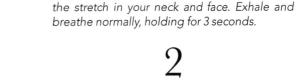

3

Place your arms under your lower back, clasping your elbows. Keep raising your chest upward and continue to point your toes.

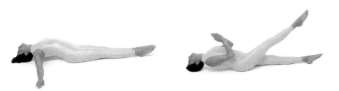

4

Inhale and raise your left leg, raising your chest. Extend your arms up with your palms together. Hold for 5 seconds. Exhale, lower your left leg, then release the neck and chest down slowly, relaxing to the floor. Hold for 10 seconds. Repeat on the other side.

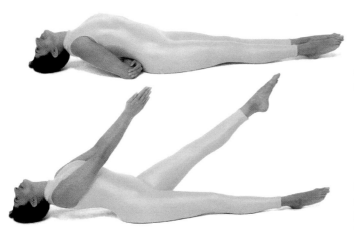

The Shoulder Stand

This is one of the most important asanas in classical yoga. Its benefits are many, the most important being that it stimulates and regulates the thyroid and parathyroid glands. Because of the chinlock, menstrual cycles regularize and weight remains stable. Healthy blood flows through the neck and chest, curing respiratory ailments and preventing sinus troubles and colds. Daily practice of this exercise cleanses the bowels and eliminates toxins.

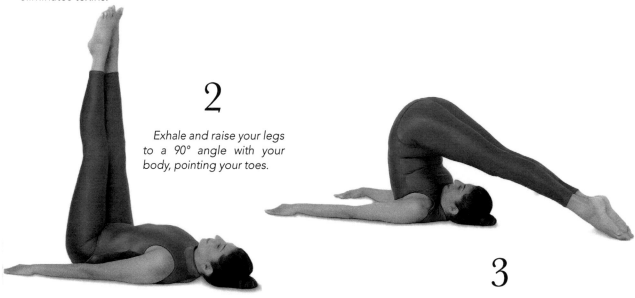

2

Exhale and raise your legs to a 90° angle with your body, pointing your toes.

3

Inhale and take your legs over your head into the Plough position. Inhale and exhale..

1

Lie flat on the floor with your arms at your sides. Inhale and bring your knees into your chest.

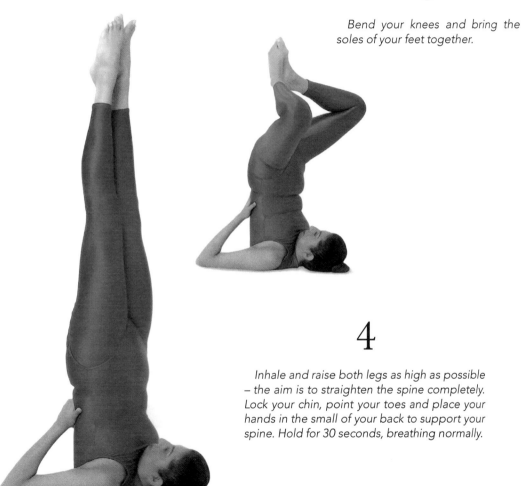

5

Bend your knees and bring the soles of your feet together.

4

Inhale and raise both legs as high as possible – the aim is to straighten the spine completely. Lock your chin, point your toes and place your hands in the small of your back to support your spine. Hold for 30 seconds, breathing normally.

The Cobra

The Cobra strengthens and tones the lower back muscles. It alleviates back pain and prevents other common back ailments. The action of The Cobra tightens the buttock muscles and increases the intra-abdominal pressure which tones the uterus and ovaries. It also regulates the menstrual cycle and helps the thyroid and adrenal glands to work more effectively.

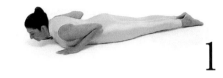

1

Lie flat on your stomach with your feet together. Point your toes, bend your arms close to your body, and place your palms flat under your shoulder blades. Point your chin downward.

2

Inhale and raise your head off the floor. Place your hands on the floor with your elbows inward. Keep your chin up and make sure your hip bones stay on the floor. Breathe normally and hold for 10 seconds. On the last exhalation, slowly lower yourself to the floor and return to Step 1. Repeat.

3

Return to Step 1, but this time place your hands under the breastbone and point your elbows outward.

4

Inhale, push down and lift your body off the floor. Look upward, keeping your shoulders down and your hips just off the floor. Breathing normally, hold for 10 seconds. On the last exhalation, slowly lower yourself and relax.

The Cat Stretch

This is a wonderful body stretch to release tension trapped in the spine. It is excellent if you are very tired, as it invigorates the nervous system and helps calm the mind. If you are experiencing any back pain this is the best way to ease it. This is a relaxed pose, so you can hold it for as long as you wish. Inhale and exhale deeply to increase the calming effect.

1

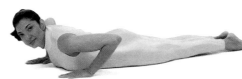

Lie flat on the floor and bend your arms, keeping your hands under your shoulder blades. Point your toes and relax your elbows, but hold them close to your body.

2

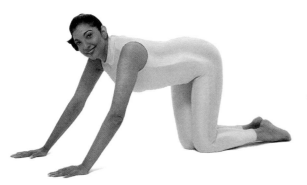

Inhale deeply and push down on your palms so that you can lift your hips upward into a kneeling position just like a cat.small of your back to support your spine. Hold for 30 seconds, breathing normally.

3

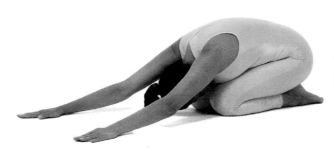

Exhale and stretch your hips back so that you sit on your heels. Straighten your elbows, stretching your arms out in front of you. Place your forehead on the floor. Breathe normally and relax.

The Camel

The Camel tones the entire spine as well as every muscle group in the body, building strength in the lower back and alleviating back ailments, especially sciatica and slipped discs. It is also a wonderful stretch for the face and neck – the increased circulation helps to prevent the signs of ageing. Every time you do this exercise, feel your body giving way into the stretch and relax and open the throat and chest; do not allow any weight into the thighs or leg muscles. Always push upward from the hips to increase the intensity of the back stretch and breathe deeply throughout. If you experience a sharp pain in the lower back, stop immediately and relax in Step 3. A dull pain means you are using muscles around the spine that need toning.

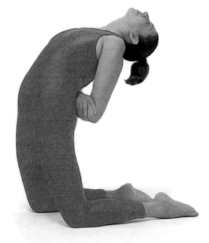

1

Kneel down, spine straight and hips directly above your knees. Hold on to your elbows behind your lower back. Inhale, push your hips forward and drop your head back. Breathe normally.

2

Continuing to push your hips forward, take your hands to your heels. Open your chest and throat and relax your face, neck and shoulders. Say 'Aah' in a clear tone to test that you are in the correct position. Breathe normally and hold for as long as possible

3

To release the spine, reverse the position by relaxing your head down to the floor with your palms facing up. Breathe normally and repeat the exercise.

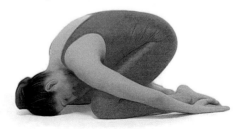

The Rabbit

The Rabbit allows fresh oxygen into the blood supply, which stimulates and invigorates the brain cells. The upside-down position of the head has a beneficial effect on the pituitary gland and thyroid. It wards off senility, clarifies the mind, regulates the metabolism and strengthens the immune system. It also has a calming effect on the nervous system. A preliminary exercise to the Head Stand (page 124), the Rabbit improves the elasticity and mobility of the spine.

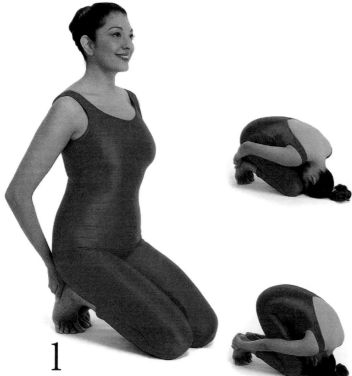

2

Inhale and as you exhale curl your spine and place your forehead on the floor as close as you can to your knees. Breathe normally.

3

Roll on to the top of your head. Straighten your elbows and raise your hips. Breathe deeply and hold for 20 seconds. Return to Step 1 and repeat the exercise.

1

Kneel on the floor, toes tucked under your haunches. Clasp your hands to your heels and sit up tall. Breathe normally.

Soles of the Feet

This Soles of Feet movement opens up the hips and increases flexibility in the hip joints, knees and thighs. Rotating the legs outward helps to increase the body's suppleness and also improves overall posture and mobility of the spine. It is an ideal exercise to do in preparation for giving birth, but take care not to bounce or jerk the spine.

1

Sit up tall on the floor with your legs in front of you. Bring the soles of your feet together and reach forward to place your hands around your ankles.

2

Bring the heels closer into your body and sit upright. Relax your shoulders, then stretch up from the pelvis and open out the chest.

3

To increase the stretch of the hips, thighs and knees, place your elbows over the knees. Bend over, curving your spine and keeping your shoulders down. Inhale, and

Sitting Twist

If you practice these twisting movements regularly, any pain that you are suffering in your lower back will rapidly diminish. The muscles of your neck will also be strengthened, especially when you look over the shoulder (not shown) and any tension is released from your spinal system. Your liver and spleen are activated by the movements and the size of your abdomen is reduced in the twisting position..

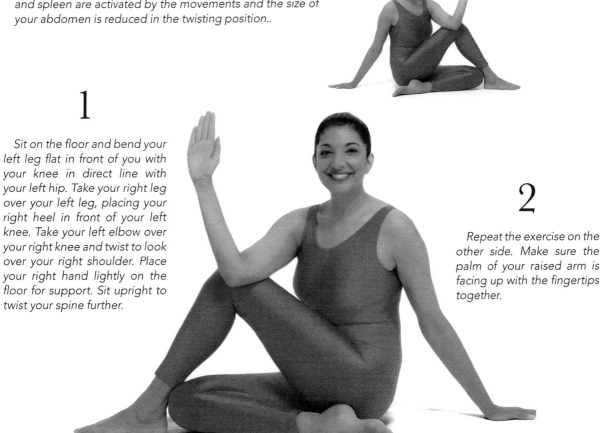

1

Sit on the floor and bend your left leg flat in front of you with your knee in direct line with your left hip. Take your right leg over your left leg, placing your right heel in front of your left knee. Take your left elbow over your right knee and twist to look over your right shoulder. Place your right hand lightly on the floor for support. Sit upright to twist your spine further.

2

Repeat the exercise on the other side. Make sure the palm of your raised arm is facing up with the fingertips together.

55

Pranayama

'Prana' is the Sanskrit word for energy and 'pranayama' is the yoga breathing technique that unblocks this flow in the body and balances the masculine and feminine energies. Breathing correctly from the diaphragm acts as a natural tranquilizer and calms the nervous system. Always breathe through the nose, and as you exhale you will find that your lung capacity is increased and that more oxygen reaches the bloodstream. This rejuvenates the blood cells and increases vitality.

1

Sit cross-legged on the floor, or on a chair with your lower back supported, in which case keep your knees together and your feet flat on the floor. Place your thumb and first finger together and turn your palms upward. Focus on your diaphragm, and try to keep one thought in your mind. Breathe deeply, holding the position for at least 60 seconds.

2

To release tension in the neck and shoulders, inhale and raise your shoulders to your ears. Then exhale and lower them again. Repeat 3 times.

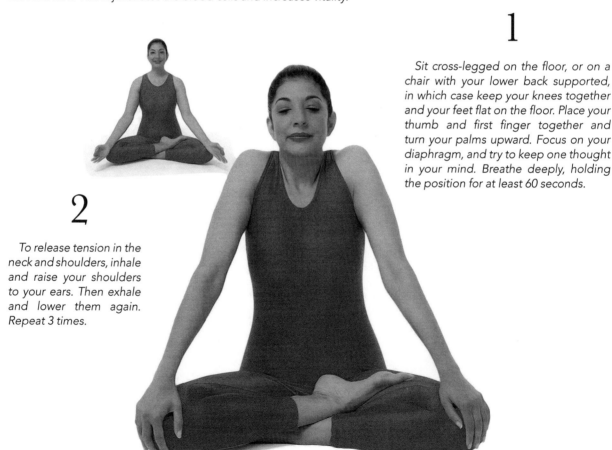

Pranayama - Meditation

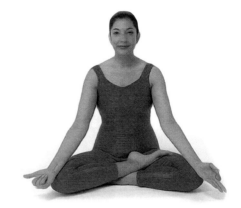

1

Sit cross-legged or in lotus or half lotus position, your spine upright. Touch your left thumb and first finger together and fold the three middle fingers of your right hand into your palm, extending your thumb and little finger.

2

Take your right hand to your nose and block the left nostril with your little finger. Inhale and exhale deeply through the right nostril only. Continue for 10 breaths.

3

Block the right nostril with your thumb and breathe for 10 seconds. Repeat the exercise 3 times on each side. Finish by breathing through both nostrils as in Step 1.

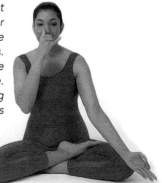

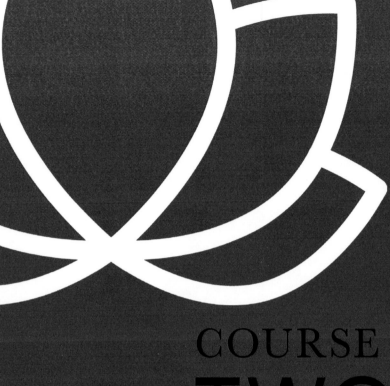

COURSE

TWO

Course Two

INTRODUCTION

By now you have become familiar with the general style of yoga exercises and you have gained more flexibility, strength and stamina. You are now ready to twist your body in various ways, remembering, of course, to start with the Warm-Up (see ABOVE).

In Course Two you will experience the energy flowing from one position to another. The muscles, joints and blood vessels will all be stretched, so that the blood is equally distributed to every part of the body and more energy flows into the relaxed muscles.

Try to hold the postures for longer with a calm and still mind. The only difference between a beginner and an intermediate student of yoga is the length of time a pose is held. This gives time for the mind to focus and the body to cleanse, purify and build the system.

Head to Knee

This Head to Knee exercise lengthens the spine forward and is an excellent way to increase your body's flexibility and release unwanted body toxins. It helps soothe the nervous system, and will also relax the brain. You should never force your body forward, but as you increase the depth of your breathing you will be able to ease into the joy of deep stretching. It is very important to stretch forward from the waist. At the same time keep your back flat and don't round your shoulders. You might feel a pull in your hamstrings or some stiffness in the lower back. If this happens and you feel a bit dizzy, stretch your spine forward halfway, put your palms on a wall and keep your feet slightly apart.

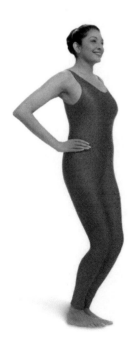

1

Begin the exercise by standing up straight. Bend your knees slightly and place your hands on your waist.

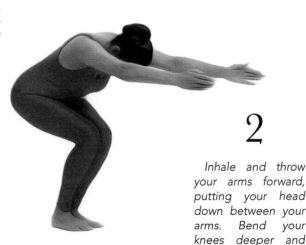

2

Inhale and throw your arms forward, putting your head down between your arms. Bend your knees deeper and keep your head in line with your back.

3

Exhale and then throw your arms out straight behind your back, in line with your shoulders, but still keep your body in the same bent position.

4

Take your hands down and hold your ankles from behind, moving your head down toward your knees. Breathe normally for 5 seconds.

5

Now straighten your knees as much as you can. Pull your stomach muscles in, and drop your head down to your knees. Hold this position for at least 5 to 10 seconds. You'll feel the energy flow in a circular motion from your toes up the spine to your head. Uncurl and relax.

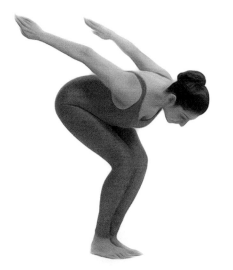

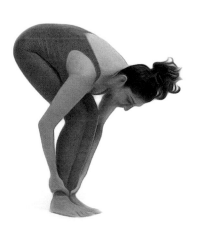

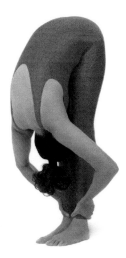

Knee Bends

These knee bend exercises build stamina and strength in the leg muscles as well as the abdominals. Balance is the key factor to doing them well, plus intense concentration. They help tone the spine as well as the calves, thighs and upper arms. The joints are also energized, which can prevent arthritis and rheumatism in the legs. These Knee Bends are grounding exercises which connect the earth's energy to the base of the spine. This energy then flows up the spine, increasing circulation and revitalizing your body.

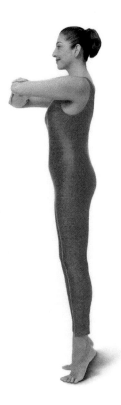

1

Stand up straight with your arms at your sides. Cross your arms in front of you and hold your elbows. Raise your heels and balance on your toes.

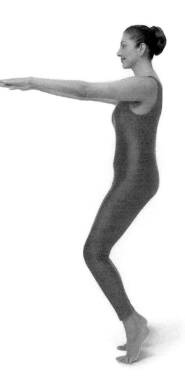

2

Straighten out your arms in front of you to help you maintain your balance. Bend your knees, keep your spine perfectly straight and try to hold still.

4

Bend right down to a squatting position. Your knees, thighs and hips should be in a line at a right angle to the floor. Breathe deeply and hold as long as you can.

3

Bend your knees down further so that you feel the extra stretch in your thighs, and keep lifting your heels upward.

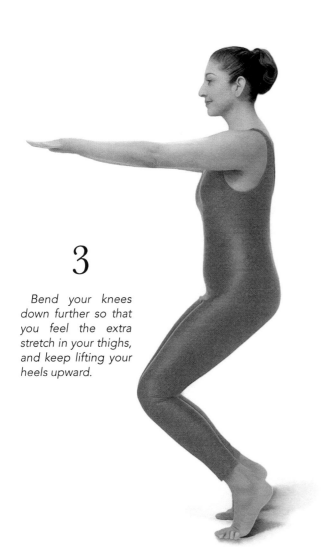

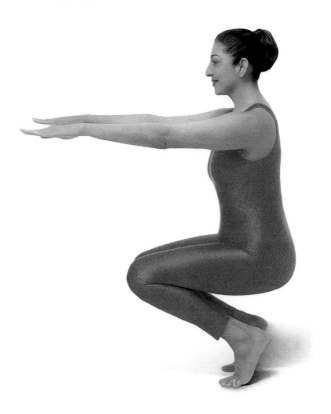

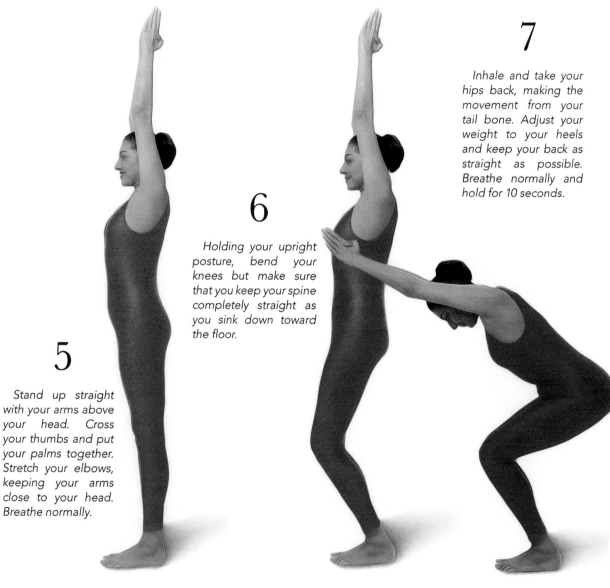

7

Inhale and take your hips back, making the movement from your tail bone. Adjust your weight to your heels and keep your back as straight as possible. Breathe normally and hold for 10 seconds.

6

Holding your upright posture, bend your knees but make sure that you keep your spine completely straight as you sink down toward the floor.

5

Stand up straight with your arms above your head. Cross your thumbs and put your palms together. Stretch your elbows, keeping your arms close to your head. Breathe normally.

Side Leg Stretch

This exercise looks simple but is in fact quite challenging. All the muscles in the legs are being toned and strengthened and suppleness is increased as you stretch to the side. The most important thing to remember is to keep the hips square. Open your chest without altering your posture and keep lifting as tall as you can. This position creates a positive attitude and the balance gives you steadiness and poise.

1

Stand up straight. Imagine a string is pulling you up from the top of the head to straighten your spine further. Put your left hand on your waist and use your right hand to lift your right leg up to the inner left thigh. Breathe normally.

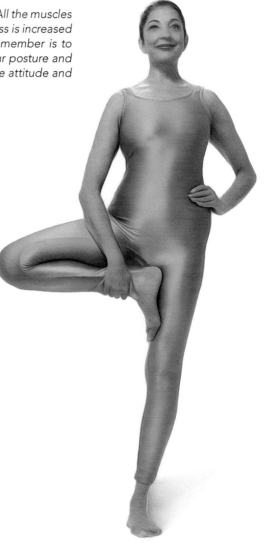

Tips

• *In all balancing exercises, keep your eyes focused on one spot as this helps to center your body and focus your mind.*

• *If your ankle wavers from side to side during this exercise, grip the floor with your toes.*

• *Do not collapse your spine forward when you clasp your toes in Step 2.*

• *If you cannot stretch your leg completely in Step 3, bend your knee.*

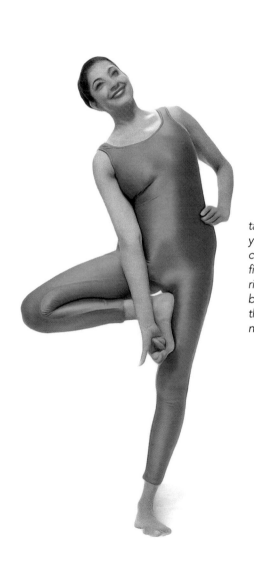

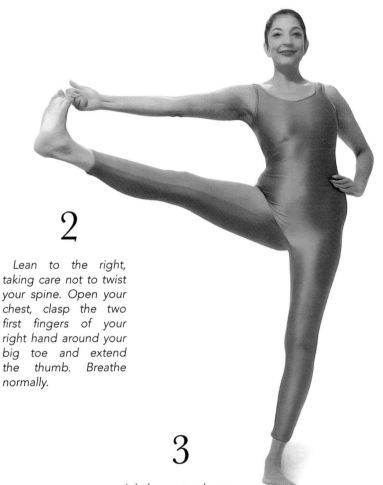

2

Lean to the right, taking care not to twist your spine. Open your chest, clasp the two first fingers of your right hand around your big toe and extend the thumb. Breathe normally.

3

Inhale, extend your right leg out from the knee and straighten your spine, taking care not to swivel your hips. Breathe normally and hold for as long as you can. Repeat on the other side.

Half-Moon

This asana conveys harmony, balance, poise and power. It will give you a sense of achievement to flow into the final pose gracefully, without jerking. Before you begin the exercise, imagine yourself in the final position and feel as if you are a dancer as you move from one step to the next. The Half Moon also strengthens and tones the leg muscles and improves concentration.

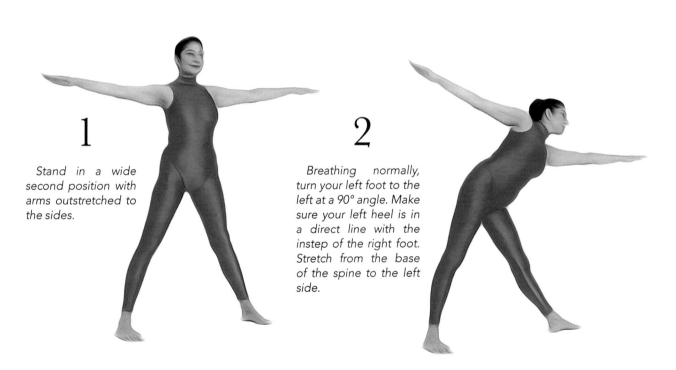

1

Stand in a wide second position with arms outstretched to the sides.

2

Breathing normally, turn your left foot to the left at a 90° angle. Make sure your left heel is in a direct line with the instep of the right foot. Stretch from the base of the spine to the left side.

3

Bend your left knee, take your right hand to your waist and place your left hand on the floor. Look straight ahead and steady your balance. Breathe normally.

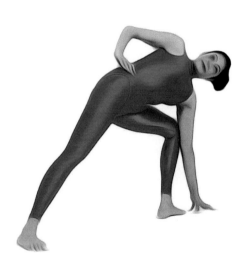

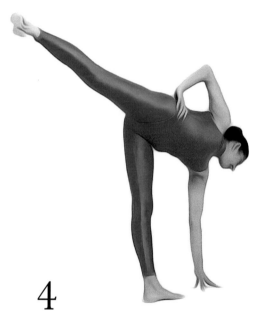

4

Focus on one spot on the floor. Inhale as you straighten your left knee and raise your right leg off the floor. Breathing normally, hold as long as possible; look over your right shoulder if you can. Repeat on the other side.

Lunge with Balance

This exercise strengthens and tones all the muscles of the legs, stomach and arms. It builds stamina and suppleness of the spine. The position of the back stimulates the heartbeat and, with the increased oxygen pumped to the lungs, rejuvenates and energizes the entire body. The aim is to increase the mind control over the body while focusing attention and concentration on the physical. It needs tremendous skill to master this exercise, so do not become discouraged if it takes some time to learn. When you are in this pose it gives you a sense of harmony, balance, poise and power. It is especially recommended for runners and dancers as it brings vigor, agility and good carriage.

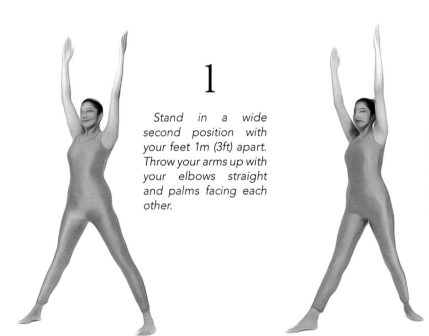

1

Stand in a wide second position with your feet 1m (3ft) apart. Throw your arms up with your elbows straight and palms facing each other.

2

Turn your right foot to the right in a 90° angle to the left foot. Make sure the right heel is in line with the instep of the left foot. Breathe normally.

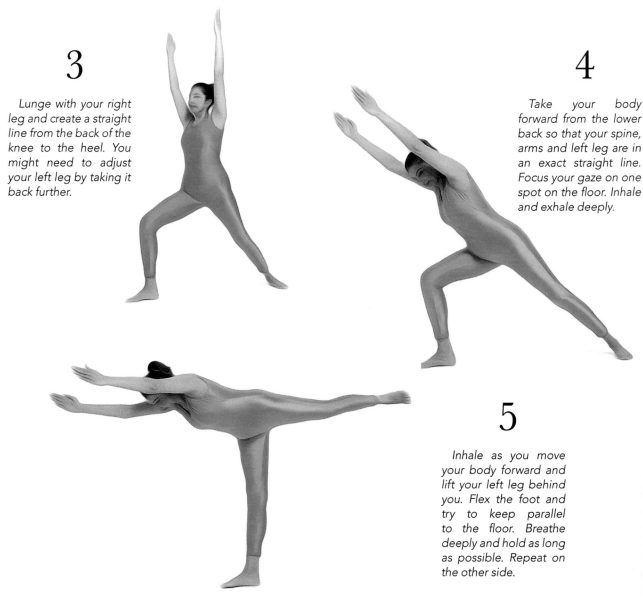

3

Lunge with your right leg and create a straight line from the back of the knee to the heel. You might need to adjust your left leg by taking it back further.

4

Take your body forward from the lower back so that your spine, arms and left leg are in an exact straight line. Focus your gaze on one spot on the floor. Inhale and exhale deeply.

5

Inhale as you move your body forward and lift your left leg behind you. Flex the foot and try to keep parallel to the floor. Breathe deeply and hold as long as possible. Repeat on the other side.

Side Lunge

This series of movements increases flexibility of the spine, improves balance and tones and cleanses the abdominal organs. You may feel dizzy or nauseous during the exercise, but this is a good sign – it means you are releasing toxins in the system. Just stop if you feel in any way uncomfortable and breathe deeply to regain your equilibrium. Always stretch from the tail bone and keep your hips and torso square to the side.

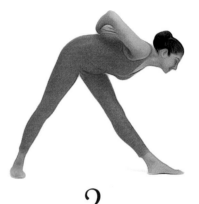

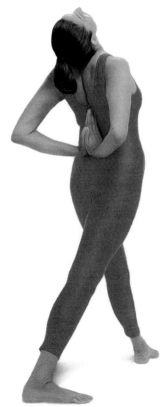

1

Follow feet positions in Steps 1 and 2 of Side Stretch (page 29). Place palms together behind your lower back or toward the mid-back. Push the elbows toward each other and open the chest. Look up and bend back as far as possible. Inhale deeply.

2

Exhale and, keeping your spine straight and your chin up, lower yourself to a 90° angle to the floor.

3

Still exhaling, bend and rest your forehead on your knee. Keep both legs straight – lift the muscles above the kneecaps to maintain balance. Breathing normally, hold for 6 seconds.

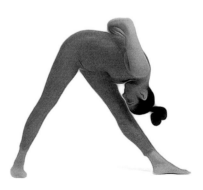

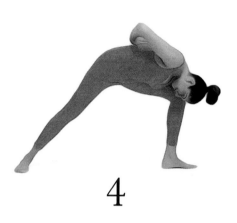

5

Straighten your knee, relax your arms down and place your hands on the floor, palms down. Breathe deeply and hold for as long as you can.

4

Bend your left knee and lunge forward. Drop your head down on the inner side of the knee. Breathe deeply and hold for 6 seconds.

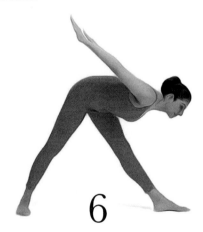

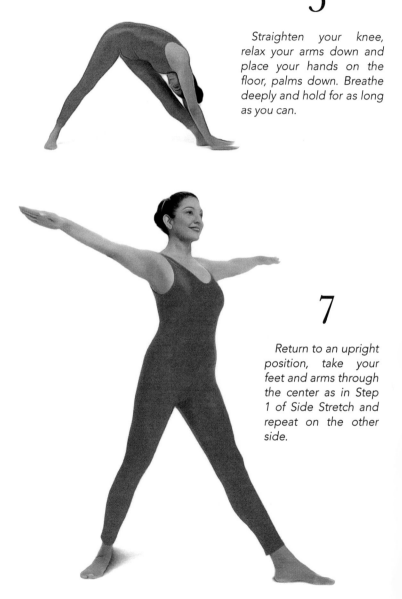

7

Return to an upright position, take your feet and arms through the center as in Step 1 of Side Stretch and repeat on the other side.

6

Inhale and raise your body so that your back is flat, with your arms back and upward. Breathing normally, hold for 6 seconds.

The Tower

This series of movements increases the strength in your legs and also makes your spine more flexible. It expands the chest, helping you to breathe more deeply and improving your lung capacity. The exercise also helps to relieve any stiffness in the neck and shoulders and make them more supple. At the end of The Tower, when your head is resting on your knee, the abdominal organs are toned and cleansed – this is because your deep breathing has pumped fresh oxygen into the blood, increasing the circulation and revitalizing and purifying them.

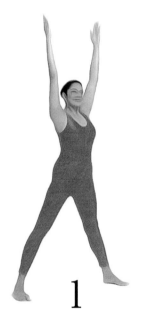

1

Stand upright with your feet about 1m (3ft) apart and your toes pointing forward. Take your arms up so that your palms face each other and straighten your elbows, keeping your shoulders down. Breathe normally.

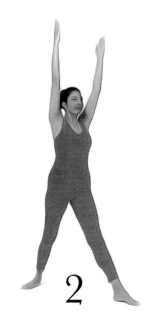

2

Turn your left foot to a 90° angle, while moving the right foot slightly inward. The heel of the left foot should be in line with your right instep. Keep your head evenly balanced between your arms.

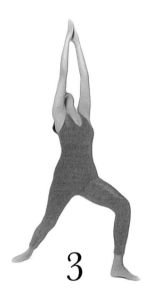

3

Bend your left leg so that your thigh is parallel to the floor. Throw your arms up and cross your thumbs with your palms together. Look upward and arch your spine. Breathe deeply and hold for 8 seconds.

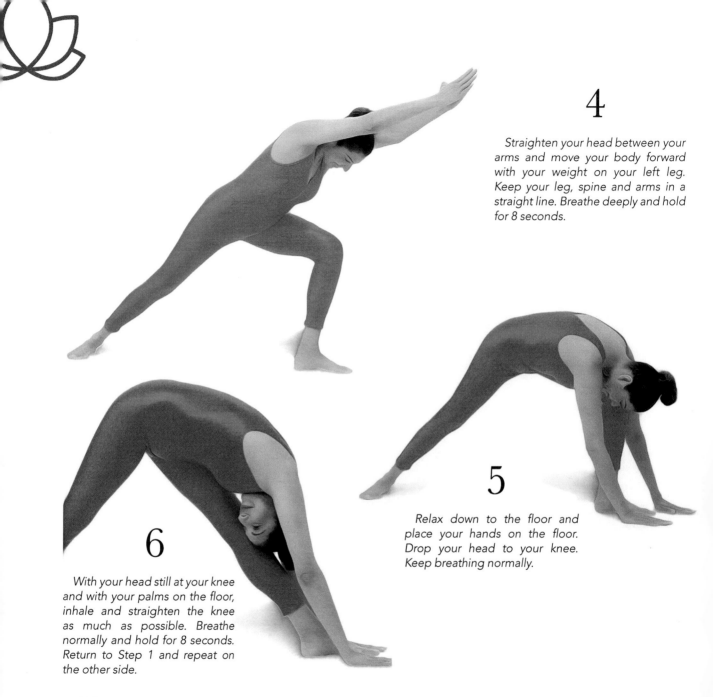

4

Straighten your head between your arms and move your body forward with your weight on your left leg. Keep your leg, spine and arms in a straight line. Breathe deeply and hold for 8 seconds.

5

Relax down to the floor and place your hands on the floor. Drop your head to your knee. Keep breathing normally.

6

With your head still at your knee and with your palms on the floor, inhale and straighten the knee as much as possible. Breathe normally and hold for 8 seconds. Return to Step 1 and repeat on the other side.

Side Stretch

Stretching to the side is an exercise that improves every muscle, joint, tendon and organ in the body. It also revitalizes the nerves, veins and body tissue by increasing the flow of oxygen to the blood. It helps cure sciatica, lumbago and other lower-back ailments. The body's strength and flexibility is heightened by the deep stretching, especially in the hip joints, waist and torso.

1

Stand up straight and place your feet about 1m (3ft) apart. Stretch out your arms with your palms facing down. Keep them in line with your shoulders. Breathe normally.

2

Turn in your left foot slightly and point your right foot 90° to the right. Inhale and stretch to the right. Keep the spine straight and do not tilt forward. Breathe normally and hold for 5 seconds.

3

Place your right hand on your right ankle and extend your left arm up in a straight line with your palm facing forward. Look up toward your arm, keeping your head up. Relax your face and shoulders, and hold for 10 seconds

4

Take the left arm over and bend to the right to feel the additional stretch. Turn your head forward and keep your weight on your back heels to maintain an equal stretch on both sides of the torso. Hold for 5 seconds.

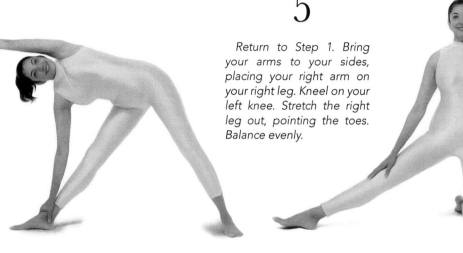

5

Return to Step 1. Bring your arms to your sides, placing your right arm on your right leg. Kneel on your left knee. Stretch the right leg out, pointing the toes. Balance evenly.

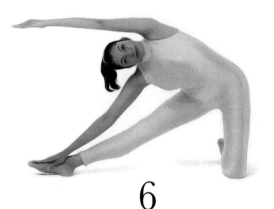

6

Inhale deeply and stretch out the right leg as far as possible without tilting forward. Stretch your left arm over to the right and feel the pull in your side. Keep your head balanced between your arms. Exhale and breathe normally.

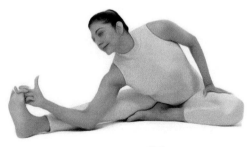

7

Now sit on the floor, stretch out your right leg and fold your left leg in front, placing your foot on your inner right thigh. Clasp your right hand around your right foot and flex your thumb. Bend your right elbow and stretch forward toward the knee.

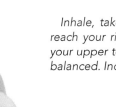

8

Inhale, take your left arm over your head and try to reach your right thumb with your fingers. Keep turning your upper torso to the side and keep your head evenly balanced. Increase the stretch and hold for 5 seconds.

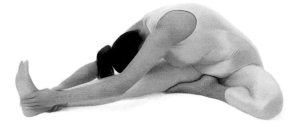

9

Exhale and relax your head and arms down over your right knee. Keep your right foot flexed and, as you breathe normally again, relax your body further down toward the floor.

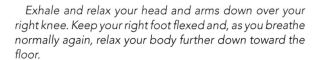

10

Lift your head up and stretch your legs out as wide as possible. Inhale and as you exhale stretch forward with your arms to reach your heels, or just reach for your thighs, knees or ankles. Stretch with your spine straight. Breathe deeply and hold for 10 seconds.

11

Now relax your head down toward the floor. Stretch your arms out, while keeping the toes flexed. Breathe normally and turn your knees upward, but push down. Hold for 15 seconds. Repeat on the other side.

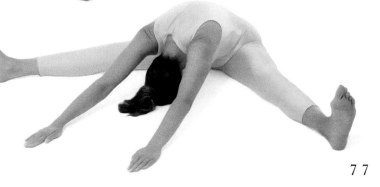

Sitting Balance

The Sitting Balance is an excellent test for checking your alignment – you will be unable to carry out this exercise if your spine is not in the correct position. Imagine your spine to be a group of children's building blocks; if you do not place each block evenly on to the next the whole building will come tumbling down. By the same token, if you do not lift your spine upright you will keep rolling back down to the floor. Concentrate on your stomach muscles because it is equally important to pull them in at the same time as you lift your spine.

1

Sit upright and bring your knees up with your feet flat on the floor. Clasp your elbows under your knees. Keep your spine straight and breathe normally.

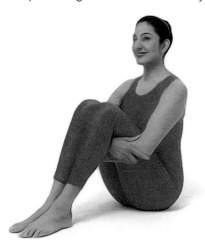

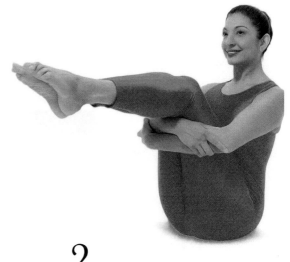

2

Still sitting upright, bring your legs up to form an exact right-angle with the body.

3

Straighten both legs up in front of you and hold the position absolutely still for at least 5 seconds, breathing normally.

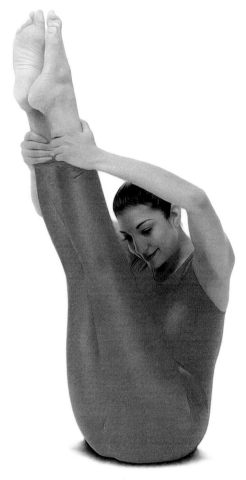

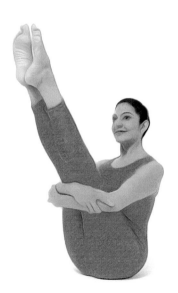

4

Shift your hands up your legs and take hold of your ankles. Pull your head toward your knees, keeping your spine straight and pulling your stomach muscles in. Breathe normally and hold for at least 5 seconds.

The Plough

This is an all-body stretch that maximizes the flexibility of the spine and tones the leg and stomach muscles. The locking of the chin into the chest stimulates the thyroid gland, which regulates the metabolism and the hormonal levels in the body. Consequently, the Plough can help to cure an overactive or underactive thyroid and stabilize weight gain and irregular menstrual cycles. This inverted position unblocks energy, improves circulation and calms the nerves. Keep your breathing deep and even to achieve maximum benefits. Do not attempt inverted postures if you are pregnant or if you have a heavy menstrual period.

1

Lie flat on the floor with your arms to the sides, palms facing down. Inhale and, using your stomach muscles, bring your knees into your chest. Keep your shoulders down and relax the muscles in your face.

2

Exhale and throw your legs behind your head to the floor. Point your toes and straighten your knees. Keep stretching your legs and lock your chin into your chest. Breathe deeply.

3

To increase the stretch, tuck your toes under and clasp your hands together. Continue to breathe deeply.

4

Holding the same position, inhale and raise your right leg straight up. Point the toes and keep both knees straight. Breathing normally, hold the position for 5 seconds. On an exhalation lower the leg slowly and repeat on the opposite leg.

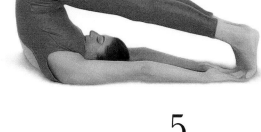

5

To release the position, take both arms and legs behind you and place your toes into your palms. Close your eyes, breathe deeply and hold for 5 to 10 seconds.

6

To relax the spine drop your knees to the floor, close to your ears. Take your arms down in front of you, palms facing down. Hold for 5 to 10 seconds.

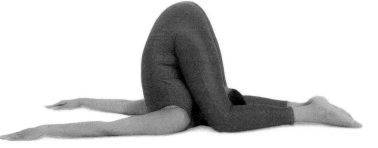

7

To begin the descent back, lift your knees off the floor and place them just above your face. Point your toes and concentrate on your spine. Breathe normally.

8

Focus on your stomach muscles and lower back and slowly straighten your legs behind you, keeping the top of your spine on the floor. Breathe normally.

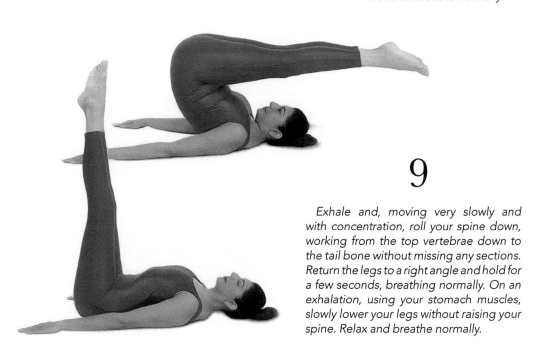

9

Exhale and, moving very slowly and with concentration, roll your spine down, working from the top vertebrae down to the tail bone without missing any sections. Return the legs to a right angle and hold for a few seconds, breathing normally. On an exhalation, using your stomach muscles, slowly lower your legs without raising your spine. Relax and breathe normally.

The Wheel

The Wheel, Bow and Camel are intense back bends that invigorate the spine, alleviate back pain and increase the lung capacity. We rarely stretch backward and these positions release fear and bestow a positive outlook on life. All three asanas release energy in the body's cells, glands and organs. The Wheel also builds muscle tone in the legs, hips, shoulders, arms, wrists and hands. Holding the position will build body strength and give stamina to the spine and limbs.

2

Keeping your feet in the same position, lift your hips and buttocks and take your arms over your head with palms facing downward. Push up and rest on the crown of your head. Breathe normally and hold for 5–10 seconds.

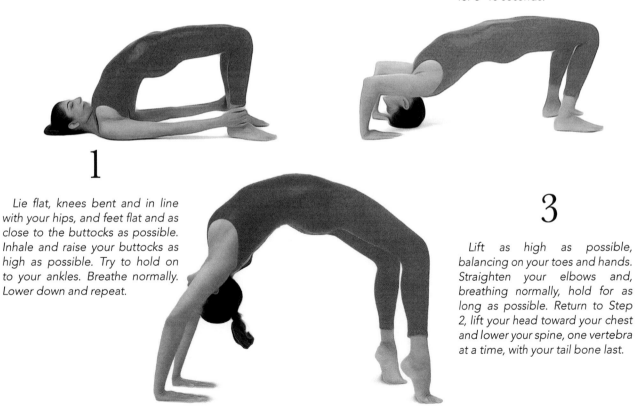

1

Lie flat, knees bent and in line with your hips, and feet flat and as close to the buttocks as possible. Inhale and raise your buttocks as high as possible. Try to hold on to your ankles. Breathe normally. Lower down and repeat.

3

Lift as high as possible, balancing on your toes and hands. Straighten your elbows and, breathing normally, hold for as long as possible. Return to Step 2, lift your head toward your chest and lower your spine, one vertebra at a time, with your tail bone last.

Back Lift

This exercise is rather strenuous to do and your body needs to be correctly aligned to achieve the right results. Not only does this type of lift tone the legs, buttocks, and stomach muscles, it also strengthens the lower back to enable you to sit and stand with perfect posture. Both your hip bones and shoulder blades should remain on the floor to stop you moving from side to side throughout the exercise. As a beginner you need not worry about the height of your leg lift, but as you gain strength and continue practicing, your hips will become more flexible and you will be able to lift your legs even higher.

1

Lie on the floor face down. Keep your back straight and place your arms by your sides, holding your hands as fists. Inhale and raise your left leg, keeping your hips square. Breathe normally and hold for 6 seconds. On the last exhalation slowly lower the leg, then inhale and repeat on the other side.

2

With your feet together, raise your hips slightly off the floor with your elbows resting under the hip bones. Keep your hands in fists, balanced under the thighs for support.

3

Inhale and raise your legs. Place your forehead on the floor. Keep lifting, breathing deeply, for as long as you can. On the last exhalation lower both legs. Repeat, then turn your head to one side and relax.

The Bow

This exercise is called the Bow because of the beautiful bow shape that the spine creates. The back muscles and internal organs are massaged and the latter invigorated. Because of the position of the abdomen, this asana helps to cure digestive and bowel disorders such as gastroenteritis and constipation. It also stimulates the appetite, aids digestion and reduces fat along the stomach and middle of the back. As a result of the increased suppleness it gives to the spine every cell in the body is rejuvenated and revitalized, giving you renewed vitality and a more youthful appearance.

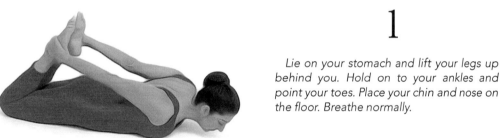

1

Lie on your stomach and lift your legs up behind you. Hold on to your ankles and point your toes. Place your chin and nose on the floor. Breathe normally.

2

Inhale and lift your body up in one movement. Balance on your hip bones and keep stretching upward, trying to get your head in line with your feet. Breathe deeply and hold for as long as you can.

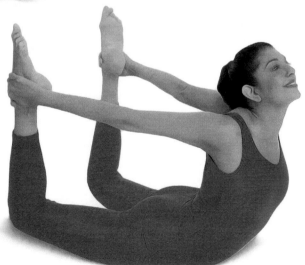

Spinal Twist

The Spinal Twist opens the hip area, increases flexibility of the spine and releases toxins from the adrenal glands. It also tones the abdominal organs, kidneys, and spleen, aids digestion and cures digestive disorders. This pose stimulates the blood circulation to the spine and relieves backache. Because the abdominal wall is being contracted the abdominal muscles are stretched on both sides. When you are in the final position you will feel invigorated and energized.

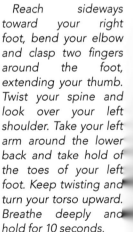

1

Sit on the floor with both legs stretched straight out in front of you. Flex your right foot and take your left leg into a half-lotus. Sit upright and try to bring your left knee down to the floor. Breathe normally.

2

Reach sideways toward your right foot, bend your elbow and clasp two fingers around the foot, extending your thumb. Twist your spine and look over your left shoulder. Take your left arm around the lower back and take hold of the toes of your left foot. Keep twisting and turn your torso upward. Breathe deeply and hold for 10 seconds.

3

Release your left arm and take it sideways over your head to touch the right thumb. Keep your head even between your arms. Breathing normally, hold for 10 seconds. Repeat on the other side.

Toe Pull

This Toe Pull exercise stretches the body forward from the hips, helps to strengthen the leg muscles and increases the flexibility of the hamstrings and the spine. The movement stimulates the kidneys, liver and pancreas as you pull in the abdominal muscles. It also helps to flatten the stomach.

1

Sit upright with your legs out in front of you. Flex both feet and raise your arms over your head. Hold onto your elbows, keeping your shoulders down. Breathe normally.

2

Bend forward from the hips, keeping the back flat. Try not to curve your spine. Hold up your chin, keeping your head balanced between your arms. Hold for 5 seconds.

3

Reach further forward and try to grasp two fingers around your big toes. Flex the thumbs and keep the elbows straight. Inhale and exhale, and hold for 5 seconds.

4

Bend your elbows and stretch forward, pointing your chin. Keep your back flat and your head out in front. Breathe deeply and hold for 10 seconds.

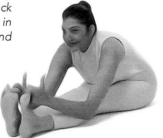

Eye Exercise

This exercise strengthens and tones the muscles in and around the eyes, increasing circulation and preventing wrinkles and fine lines from forming. It is also called the Clock because in doing it you visualize the numbers of a clock in clockwise and counter-clockwise fashion. Do not move your head but exaggerate the movement of your eyes. You may experience some strain but this is due to weak eye muscles; rub your hands together to make them warm and then cup your eyes to rest them. The shoulder stretch is optional, but it is a good companion to the eye stretch.

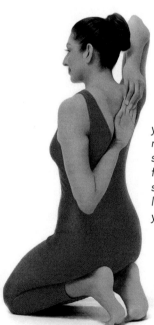

1

Kneel on the floor, tucking your toes under. Take your right arm over your right shoulder, placing your palm face down between your shoulder blades. Take your left arm around and clasp your hands together.

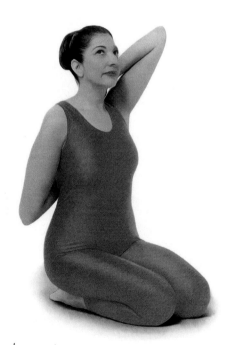

2

Keeping your chin level, look up at the number 12 of an imaginary clock. Focusing on each number, move your eyes clockwise, then repeat counter-clockwise. Repeat the exercise on the other side.

Total Stretch

This stretch is very controversial – some people find it excruciating, while others feel it to be the most marvelous of all the classic stretches. The truth is that the more flexible you are the easier the pose. It stretches every muscle in the thighs, knees and ankles, as well the entire spine. If you feel any pain in your back, place a pillow under the small of the back and open your chest. If you feel your knees are strained place a small pillow under the back of your knees. The most important thing to remember is to relax in the position. Breathe deeply and evenly and feel the chest and hips open.

1

Sit upright and bring your knees together. Spread your feet and rest them either side of your hips, with your buttocks on the floor. Place your palms facing forward on your feet.

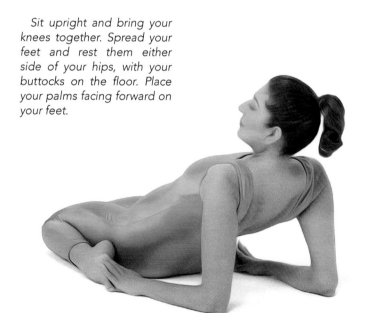

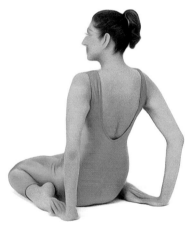

2

Drop your body back down, taking your weight on your elbows, and feel the stretch in your legs and abdomen.

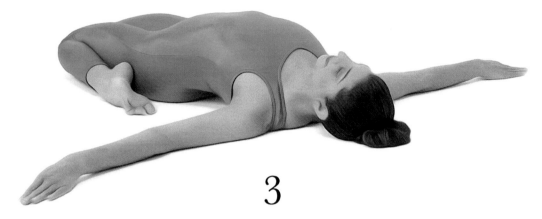

3

Lie back flat on the floor with your arms stretched out to the sides.

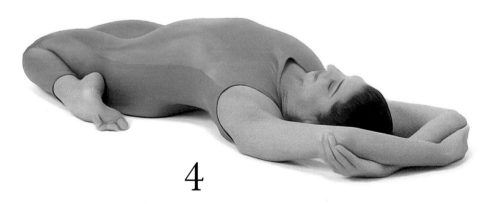

4

Clasp your elbows. Continue to breathe deeply and relax the entire body and mind. Try to hold this position for as long as possible – with practise you will be able to sustain it for 10–15 minutes.

Uddiyana

In Sanskrit, 'Uddiyana' means 'flying up'. In this exercise the air is drawn up from the lower abdomen and moves under the ribcage toward the head. This movement tones the abdominal organs, increases the gastric juices and eliminates toxins in the digestive tract. It is a wonderful way to exercise the muscles of the stomach, thereby making it flatter.

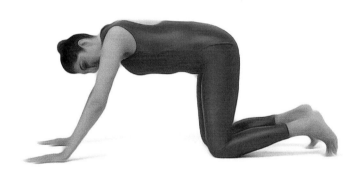

1

Kneel down on all fours. Keep your spine straight and place your hands and feet in a direct line. Inhale through your nose and exhale through your mouth until all the breath is out of your lungs.

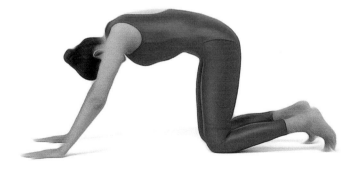

2

Pull the stomach muscles up and curve your spine slightly. Without taking a breath, contract and release the muscles to massage the internal organs. When you tire, inhale and exhale normally for a few breaths. Repeat the whole exercise up to 20 times.

QUICK FIXES FOR COMMON AILMENTS

Quick Fixes for Common Ailments

Yoga plays an integral part in helping prevent medical disorders. This branch is called Remedial Yoga when a practioner prescribes certain asanas to alleviate pain and build the immune system.

It is now possible to prove scientifically the effect of remedial yoga, and clinical trials have shown its beneficial results. In the past we had to rely on the Yogis who believed that Yoga is a holistic approach to physical and mental wellness. In the ancient texts, it explicitly describes which exercises work on specific organs, nerves, especially the brain. We are now ,with scientific evidence, able to measure which cells are stimulated and many physicians are now prescribing Yoga to their patients as an anecdote to stress relief. There are four phases of stress disorders. The first is the physic phase. The symptoms are irritability, energy loss, sleeplessness, and anxiety attacks. If unchecked, the person moves to the second, psychosomatic phase and experiences hypertension, tremors, or palpitations. The next phase is the somatic phase when illness develops in the vital organs. The fourth phase is the organic phase when the organ is in full-fledged inflammatory change. Medical attention is now required.

Yoga can help prevent the first stage, relieve the symptoms of the second phase, develop a therapy programmed for the third, and with modern medicine help the body to restore its natural equilibrium in the fourth phase.

Remedial Yoga takes the physical disorder and applies a specific exercise that will alleviate the symptoms, or a series of exercises to help cure the ailment

Here are a few fixes for our Chronic Ailments.

Arthritis

This is an excellent way to relieve stiffness in the joints, especially in the feet, hands, knees, hips and shoulders. In the beginning this exercise might feel uncomfortable but continued practice will alleviate the pain and increase circulation to the joints.

Kneel up tall then tuck the toes under and sit back on the heels. If you feel any pain release the toes and continue with the exercise. Place the hands behind you for support, fingers pointing away from you. Keep your arms and spine straight. Breathing normally, lift your hips up and push them forward as high as possible while balancing on your hands. Your weight should be evenly distributed between your arms and hips. Drop your head back, lifting your chin and hips up to create a circular pattern with your spine. Hold for at least 5 seconds and repeat. When you are able to hold this pose comfortably increase to 10 seconds.

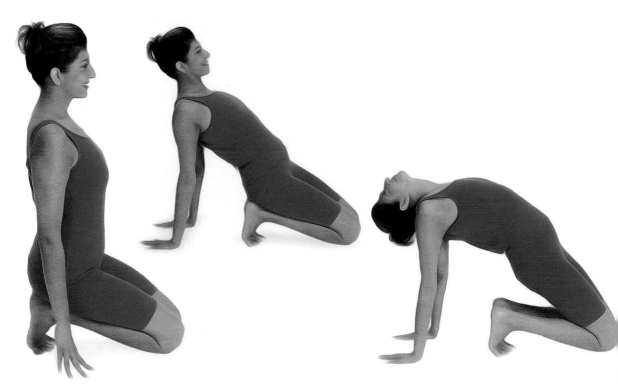

Osteoporosis

As you age it is vital to take extra calcium to stop the bones from becoming brittle. Equally important in preventing this condition from occurring is keeping a fresh blood supply to the hip area. This twist sends fresh oxygen and a purified blood supply to the hips and increases the circulation of the entire system. It alleviates painful conditions like sciatica as well as strengthing the hip joints.

Stand tall with your feet 1-1.2m (3-4ft) apart. Turn your left foot to the left and make sure your left heel is in a direct line with the instep of your right foot. Take your arms out to the side in line with your shoulders. Bend your right elbow so it is line with your left knee.

Inhale, put your right hand on the floor, exhale, twist your spine and look up over your left shoulder. Breathe deeply and hold for 5-7 seconds. Keep your arms in a straight line. If you are unable to touch the floor with your hand hold any part of your left leg. Repeat on the other side.

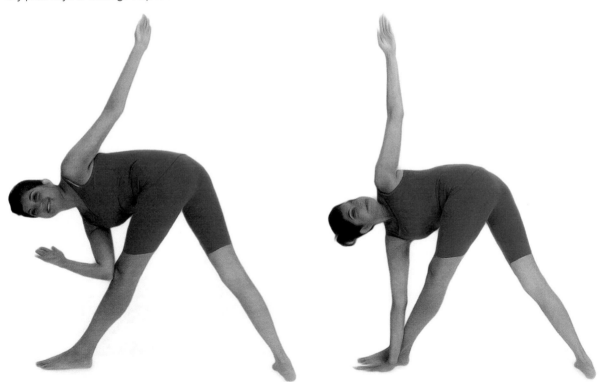

Immune System

When the immune system is weak the body is vulnerable to all kinds of health issues and problems. Many factors weaken the immune system especially stress and emotional trauma. Even though we cannot eliminate stress from our daily lives we can learn to boost the immune system in order to prevent ailments from becoming chronic.

Sit sideways on the floor, leaning on your right hip. Straighten your right leg and point your toe. Take your left knee up so your left foot is flat on the floor behind the right knee. Place your right palm on the floor about 30 cm (1 ft.) from your right hip. Place your left hand near the upper thigh of your right leg.

Inhale and push yourself up, balancing on your right hand and right foot. Exhale, keeping the legs parallel and your right arm fully extended. Your left arm should be pointed straight up in the air in line with your right arm. Breathe deeply and hold for as long as you can. Repeat on the other side

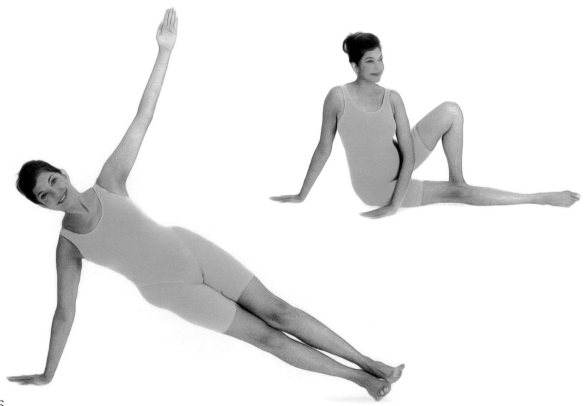

Insomnia

People who are unable to relax often find it very difficult to sleep at night. This pose allows every muscle and nerve to relax, and combined with deep breathing, will de-stress the entire nervous system. The most important thing is to relax the mind by concentrating on the breathing. Breathe from the diaphragm through the nose deep and evenly.

Kneel down on the floor so you are sitting on your heels. Leave your knees together, take your heels apart and sit down on the floor between your heels. Place your palms down on the floor, fingers touching your toes. Slowly bend your elbows and lower your body down towards the floor. Keep your head forward and feel the intense stretch in your knees and hips. Only when you are comfortable in this position proceed further down until your whole spine is on the floor. If you find this difficult place some soft pillows under the small of the back to support the spine. Take your arms over your head, hold on to your elbows and relax for as long as you feel comfortable. You will find that with continued practice this pose becomes easier to master.

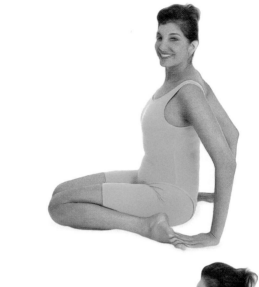

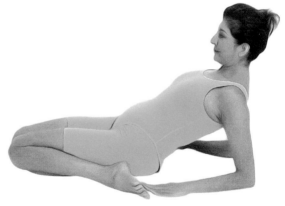

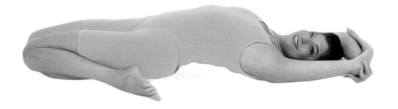

Depression

Our mental state affects us physically, so it is vital to keep a positive outlook on life. With the challenges of modern living this is not always easy. Keeping the mind alert and body mobile will prevent depression. When you are in this inverted position the blood rushes to the brain and nourishes the cells. This helps to keep the mind clear and focused.

Kneel on the floor, tuck your toes under and sit back on your heels. Interlace your fingers, make a triangle with your arms and place your elbows on to the floor. Make sure your elbows are directly in line with your shoulders. This forms your base Place the top of your head on the floor, fingertips touching the back of your head. Inhale; straighten your legs and balance on your toes. Exhale, push your shoulders down and straighten your spine. Breathing normally, hold for 5 seconds. Bend your knees to the floor. Hold for 5 seconds and repeat, this time holding for 10 seconds. Sit back on your heels, your forehead on the floor. Relax for a few moments and lift your head slowly to avoid any dizziness.

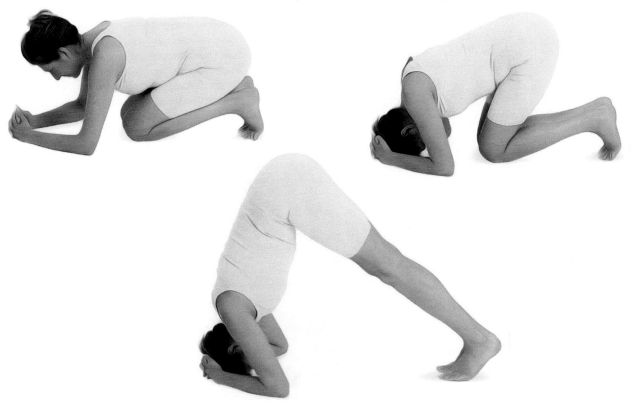

Eye Strain

As people age the eye muscles become lax. In our computer driven age, our eyes feel the strain with the glare of computer screens and hand held devices. This combination tires the eyes and vision can be impaired. This exercise strengthens and tones the eyes as well as sharpens our focus.

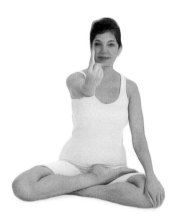

Sit up tall in a comfortable cross-legged position. Straighten your index finger of the right hand and place it in front of your nose. Stretch your arm out in front of you and stare at your finger for 5 seconds. Keeping your eyes focused on your finger, slowly bring it back towards you until it touches the tip of your nose. Still keeping your eyes focused on your finger, stretch the arm out again. Your vision might blur slightly but keep focused as this will clarify and improve your eyesight.

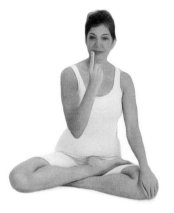

Rub your palms together to create heat and place them over your eyes. This helps to soothe and relax the eyes,

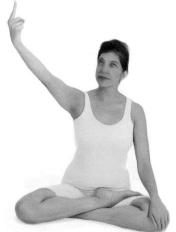

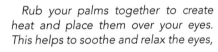

Keeping your head straight take your right arm to the right, eyes always focused on the finger. Then take your arm diagonally to the left. Repeat on the same side, then on the other side. Finish by rubbing the palms together and cup them again over your eyes.

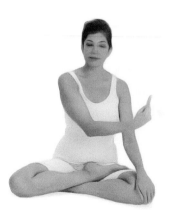

Pelvic Floor

After childbirth and advancing years, many women suffer from incontinence and other urinary disorders. The pelvic floor must be kept toned in order for the urinary system and sexual organs to function properly. As you do this exercise, contract the pelvic muscle to bring elasticity to the vaginal wall, which will increase sensation during sexual intercourse.

Lie face down on the floor, arms to the side. Place your elbows under the shoulder blades with your palms face down and your fingertips together. Inhale; push your palms and elbows down as you lift your head up. Make sure your hipbones remain on the floor Exhale and point your toes. Breathing normally, lift both legs behind you. Keeping your feet together. Balancing on your right arm, reach back with your left hand and take hold of your left foot. Lift your spine and look upwards. Hold for 5-7 seconds. Repeat on the other side.

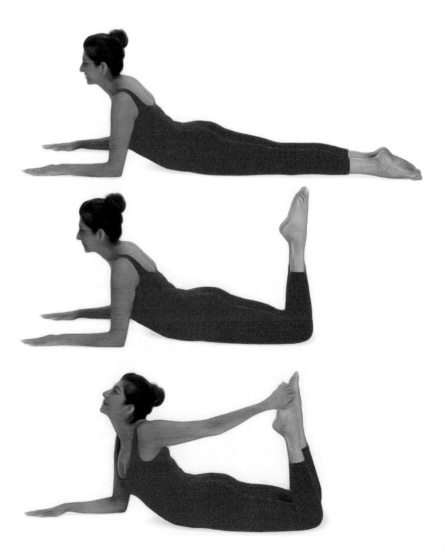

Breaks & Fractures

With advancing age, old breaks and fractures can cause arthritic conditions. This simple twist greatly improves circulation and all past injuries will receive a fresh supply of blood which will help ease the pain and boost healing.

Sit on the floor, your legs stretched out in front of you. Bring your left knee up and hold on to your leg. Breathing normally, place your right hand on the floor behind you and gently twist your body to the right so you are looking over your right shoulder. Straighten your left arm, point your fingers and keep both hipbones down on the floor as you increase the stretch.

Sit up tall, take your right hand behind your lower back with your palm facing forward, reach your left around your left knee and clasp your hands together. Keep your shoulders down as you increase the twist. Breathing deeply, hold for 7-10 seconds. Repeat on the other side.

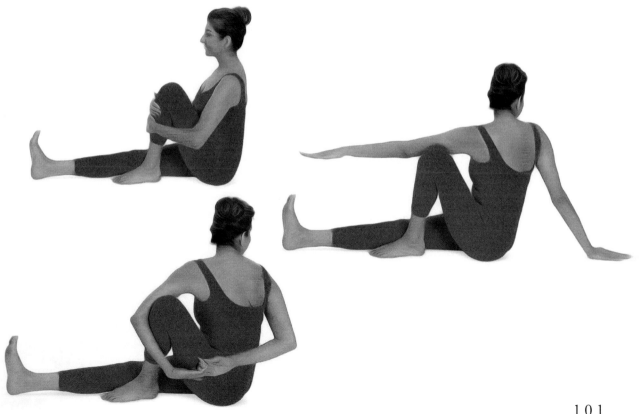

Thyroid

The thyroid is the most important gland in the body second to the pineal gland that occupies the space between the eyebrows often called the third eye. It governs the hormonal balance during your life. At different phases of life such as puberty, pregnancy, or the menopause, hormonal levels shift, causing emotional reactions and mood swings. Premenstrual syndrome is, in fact, more common today due to modern stress levels. Hormone replacement helps, but can have harmful side effects. This Yoga pose naturally relieves the imbalance and stabilizes the hormone levels. According to ancient texts, the movement of locking the chin in to the chest stimulates the thyroid. This is called an inverted posture. Do not attempt this if you are pregnant as the movement of taking your legs over your head alters the position of the uterus.

Lie flat on the floor with legs outstretched. Inhale and bring the knees in to the chest. Exhale, push your palms down to the floor and roll your legs over your head. Breathe normally and hold your lower back to support your weight. Take your knees to the floor on either side of your head close to your ears. Tighten your tummy muscles, place the soles of your feet together and create a triangle with your legs. Inhale and straighten your legs. Tighten your buttocks muscles and point as high as you can trying to keep the spine straight. Breathing deeply, hold for 20 to 30 seconds. To release, slowly bend your knees toward your forehead. Lower your spine, pushing each vertebra slowly down to the floor. Lower your legs to the floor and relax for 60 seconds.

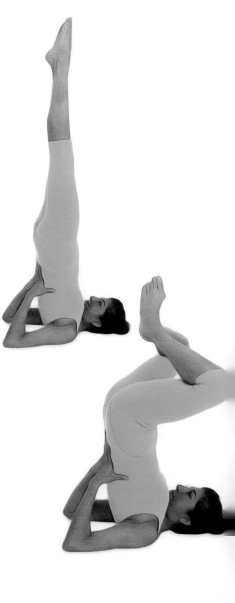

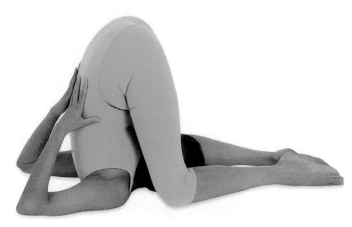

Digestive

Nervous tension in the stomach produces acidity, which can lead to gastric disorders such as flatulence, heartburn, and irritable bowel syndrome. This toxic buildup starts to eat up the stomach lining, creating imbalances. People suffering from stomachaches are often emotionally upset. The stomach muscles can seize up with muscle cramps and most people take medication to ease the pain. This simple exercise helps alleviate the pain and combined with deep breathing relaxes the stomach muscles. This helps to neutralize the stomach lining and release gases from the bowel and digestive tract.

Lie flat on the floor and point you toes. Clasp you hands behind your neck. Inhale and simultaneously lift your head and legs up in a 90-degree angle. Exhale breathe normally and hold for 5-10 seconds. Clasp your arms around your legs, holding on to the elbows. Tuck your forehead down to your knees. Point your toes and hold the position for 10 seconds. Slowly lower your spine to the floor and relax your legs down Repeat the exercise and hold for 20 seconds, breathing deeply and evenly.

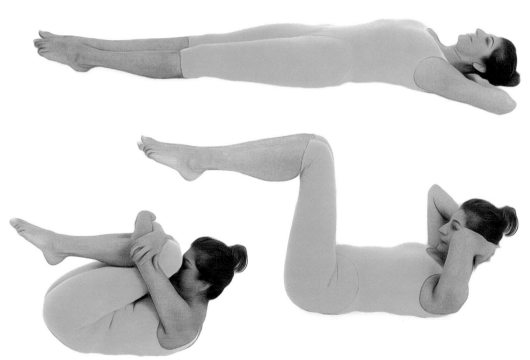

SPIRITUAL MINDFULNESS

Spiritual Mindfulness

Only raising one's consciousness can put you in the perfect flow of the universe.

Imagine a world when each and every aspect of nature and man is in perfect harmony and balance. If every person on earth practiced Yoga and connected to their higher self, we would be in a different place.

Gone the poverty that plagues the world, the oppressive government and regimes that torture their own people. Wars would not exist, only peace and happiness.

I know this sounds like an impossible film script, but this state of harmony is possible.

How do we create this paradise on earth?

Yoga philosophy teaches us that unless we are happy within ourselves, it is impossible to create loving relationships with anyone else.

We must love and take care of ourselves in order to rise to our highest level of consciousness.

When you treat yourself with love, honor, and respect, it has a magical alchemical effect on your body and your life. Every cell records the positive energy you are sending to yourself. It impacts on your DNA and changes, even deeply held beliefs and patterns. This leads you to attract other high frequency people in to your life. This keeps you happy and healthy and on the path towards your destiny.

As innocent babies and young children we are vibrating on a high dimension of frequency. As we get older and experience life's challenges we move into a lower dimension. Only when we practice spiritual techniques does our vibration rise again.

It is vital for one's soul to master the art of meditation in order to connect to the massive universal consciousness of divine light.

Your light is the energy of your soul or your divine spark radiating through you. Then you are illuminated with joy, clarity, love, wisdom, knowledge, and feelings.

Light is the frequency of your cells and how they radiate as your aura, or electromagnetic field that surrounds every person.

How do you start this process?

The most important key is Desire. You have to want it. When people begin Yoga and finally learn to master the asana, there is a sudden split second when you feel deeply connected to a spiritual source. This moment hounds you, as you want to feel this sensation again and again. At this level every physical, mental, emotional, and spiritual energies are united. It is this feeling of elation and joy that spurns you on.

Mindfullness is a big buzzword today but it really is the same as meditation, the slowing down of the mind to pay attention to one's thoughts and inner desires.

It is in this state of mind that you become acquainted with yourself and discover who you really are and what you really want.

When you learn to meditate, a whole new world becomes open to you. You begin to see the world in a totally different light. Everything seems possible. This new vista of vision propels you to a different level of consciousness. You begin to see the integration of man and nature. You see the good in all humanity. You spread the love energy to each and every soul you interact with. In other words, you see the world as totally ONE WITH THE COSMOS. You meet angels, ascendant masters, and your guardian angels in your dreams. You begin to understand the keys of the universe and your soul's place within it.

VISUALISATIONS
AND
MEDITATIONS

Visualisations and Meditations

VISUALIZATIONS AND MEDITATIONS

When you learn mind control, it is extraordinary what you can achieve by focusing your thoughts from your heart to gain what you wish to achieve in your life.

Most people do not believe that this is possible as they harbor a negative belief system.

For them they cannot think or believe that the possibilities are endless. They think there is some sort of gimmick or trick to achieving one's dreams.

This is far from the truth. When you truly open your heart and ask for what you are seeking you will be astonished at the quick results

This is the Power of Thought, a belief that you can transform your direct conversations with your subconscious mind to create reality. The first step to this change is to become aware of your thought patterns. Look at them objectively and consider whether your habits and routine prevent you from moving forward.

The second most important Law is the Power of Now. Yesterday is already a dream. It is gone and only a memory remains,

Tomorrow is only a vision yet to be fulfilled.

But today well-lived makes every yesterday a dream of happiness and every tomorrow a vision of hope.

Meditation is the key to change and transformation of one's life. When you push all the external thoughts out of your mind and visualize your life as you wish it to be, the brain cannot distinguish the difference so the visual becomes the reality. It is your own mind that is holding you back. When you alter your brain waves with real intent, you will see the changes in your life.

CANDLE GAZING

The very best way to begin training the mind is to practice the art of Candle Gazing.

Sit crossed leg with a straight spine.

Place a lit candle in front of you

With a relaxed gaze continue to look at the candle. Observe how the light flickers,

After 5-10 seconds close your eyes and you will see the flicker in the third eye. It will soon disappear.

Repeat the exercise again each time trying to prolong the image in your mind.

In the beginning, it will seem difficult to maintain the image in your mind but with continued practice the light will remain.

This forces the mind to concentrate on one thought: which is to see the flame in your third eye. The key is to hold it there for as long as possible.

This is the first stage of Meditation

VISUALIZATION OF ABUNDANCE

Find a quiet place to relax

Light a candle and/ or play soothing music.

Sit up tall with an erect spine

Begin with deep breaths from the diaphragm to calm and soothe the brain

Visualize your dream and ask the universe to fulfill this vision

Say " LIGHT THE PATH WHICH WILL LEAD ME TOWARDS AN OPPORTUNITY FOR I AM CAPABLE OF SUCCESS AND ACHIEVEMENT

BRIGHTEN MY CHANCES FOR FORTUNATE HAPPENINGS AND LIGHT THE WAY TOWARD A MORE PROMISING

FUTURE

THIS LIGHT WILL SHOW ME THE WAY I NEED TO DIRECT MY EFFORTS SO THAT I MAY SECURE THE FUNDS I NEED TO MEET MY OBLIGATIONS

THIS WILL ENRICHEN MY LIFE AND MY FAITH IS COMPLETE

Slowly turn your attention to your breath and reawaken your senses

Know where you are in time and space.

Slowly open your eyes and breathe normally

This Mantra will alter your buddhi or thoughts to success and abundance.

CHAKRA HEALING

Ayurveda Doctors believe that we have the power to heal ourselves through positive intention and cell rejuvenation.

Knowing your body intuitively and understanding its unique genetic makeup is vital to maintaining good health.

Many years ago a Yoga student recommended a book about nutrition that is called

Eat for your Blood Type. I was quite fascinated with the notion and set out to find how my blood type correlated to this Dr. theory.

I was not surprised to discover that I was eating exactly what was recommended for me.

People who practice Yoga regularly are in tune with their digestive system and intuitively know what can be digested and what nutrients are required to keep the immune system strong.

When you begin practicing Yoga, you will be surprised that your body begins to reject certain foods. Yoga does not ask you to change your diet or be vegetarian but you will discover a change in the foods that you crave.

Yoga is about moderation and finding that balance in every aspect of your life including health.

Chakras are swirling forms of energy that revolve in circles around the 7 main energy centers in the body. We call this Prana. The Chinese call this Chi and the ancient Hawaiians call it Mana.

Each chakra symbolizes a different color so in this visualization fabric or crayons make it easier to manifest the color in your mind. The purpose of this Visualization is to unblock this vital energy so that it flows steadily through the spine. I like to use the analogy of a hosepipe. If there are kinks in the pipe the water will not flow freely and only a trickle of water will result at the other end.

This correlates to a healthy spine, If these blockages are severe so this energy cannot flow fully through the system, the person will become lethargic and if vital organs are depleted of energy, dysfunction and disease will set in.

This exercise will heal and cleanse the aura, build the immune system, and prevent Illness.

Lie back on the floor in the Relaxation pose or Savasana. Palms are facing upwards and legs relaxed with feet apart.

Breathe very deeply through the nose from the diaphragm. Relax every muscle of your body beginning with the feet.

And when you feel as if you are floating on a cloud see a rainbow in your mind. Each Chakra represents a color of the rainbow so envision this spectrum of color in your mind. In order to heal the body we want the colors to be clear not cloudy. They can vary daily depending on your mental, physical, emotional, and spiritual self.

Now, focus on the color red. This represents the root chakra which is located at the

very base of the spine or Coccyx. This symbolizes survival and self-preservation.

As you inhale and exhale, focus that this energy field is healthy and whole.

Moving upwards to the second chakra visualize the color orange which symbolizes procreation and creativity. It is located below the navel. Surround your body and bathe in this light.

Yellow is the color of the solar plexus. As you inhale through the nose the universal energy enters the third chakra and then moves upwards through the spine to the crown chakra in a circular pattern to the root and second chakra. This revolving of energy takes place on each and every breath. This symbolizes self-empowerment and self-respect.

The heart chakra is symbolized by the color green. This chakra opens the heart to the concept of universal love. It invokes compassion for all of nature and sentient beings. Many people who are emotionally vulnerable walk through life with stooped shoulders with eyes cast down to protect themselves.

We need to be courageous and open our hearts to all of mankind. In this visualization green unlocks the power of love. It is the symbol of forgiveness.

As you inhale and exhale open your heart and feel the love spread. Don't be surprised if you begin to smile, as this energy is a powerful force. We must learn to love ourselves before we are able to spread this love to others.

Communication rules the fifth chakra. It is located in the throat. People who struggle to voice their opinions need to visualize the color blue, which heals and protects. As you concentrate on this energy field, feel free and emancipated that your thoughts will be heard.

Indigo rules the third eye. This is the space between the eyebrows. In meditation we learn to turn the eyes inwards towards the nose while focusing our attention to this space. An afflicted 6th Chakra represents difficulty with eyesight, cataracts, and visual impairment. As you focus on the third eye visualize your inner vision, the connection to your spiritual self. This symbolizes intuition and opens the pineal gland to the inner world of self-realization.

The 7th Chakra is the Crown, which rests at the top of the head. The color here is Violet. This represents brain function w.hich controls the entire nervous system. This chakra connects to the cosmic consciousness and universal truth. This is the unifying energy of oneness and spirituality.

Continue to inhale and exhale and feel as if you are floating on a cloud. As you float visualize a white light that envelops your entire body. This light seals and protects your aura.

Slowly return to know where you are in time and space.

Breathe normally and reflect on the experiences.you had during this exercise.

REAL YOGA

SELF-REALIZATION THROUGH YOGA

Yoga is not a religion, but a philosophy of life that brings harmony and joy to each individual. There is so much suffering in this world, yet when you understand the true reality of existence, the pain subsides and a new awareness emerges.

Everyone has a soul, yet most people

are separated from their inner self. True thoughts, wishes, and passions are ignored because of a lack of attention to what the soul needs for fulfillment. This disconnection between the soul and the physical body can manifest into illness, depression, and lack of purpose in life.

Life should be full of joy and fulfillment, no matter what obstacles arise. We are not given challenges we cannot overcome. It is these tests that build inner strength and courage, wisdom, and power to move forward. Yoga philosophy states that these lessons are given for a karmic reason. Karma is one of the Spiritual Laws that govern the Universe. It states that every Action has a Reaction or Cause and Effect.

It means that every thought, every word, every action is recorded in the Agasha or black box which then determines the circumstances that occur in this lifetime.

It makes everyone aware that the responsibility is on each individual, not blamed on others such as parents, friends, colleagues or even God when things go wrong. It shifts the thinking process to own up to one's own positive and negative thoughts and action. We say in Yoga; Be careful what you think because once action is taken the deed is done. It cannot be taken back and there will be consequences good or bad. These lessons are not given to destroy the weak, but are meant to build our inner core to the REAL understanding of the universe. That is to realize that we are all One, a part of the Divine universe. It is to know that this universe is eternal-with no beginning or end, an everlasting cycle or wheel of life governed by an all-encompassing divine source of love.

Conclusion

CONCLUSION

There are no accidents in the universe. Each and every thing that occurs has a reason. The very fact that you are reading this book already means that you are seeking change which will lead to change. It is our attitude that needs to change. When we see ourselves as part of an infinite universe your priorities will also change. When there is true connection to the inner realm through asana, pranayama, and meditation, there will be a spark of a new awareness that will shine through. When your chakras and energy field are balanced, your cells are replenished and rejuvenated and when your mind is calm and in control, you will radiate an inner glow. It never ceases to amaze me when I see a student for the first time grasp that inner light. This glow uplifts their mind and spirits. It makes all my years of teaching worthwhile just to glimpse that split second.

When the student pursues this goal, it becomes more powerful each time.

Imagine if all people on this planet practiced Yoga, what a different world would we see. Imagine my dream when all humanity is one and when everyone is happy and fulfilled; a world free of conflict and despair, a world without poverty and injustice. I truly believe this to become a reality once people change their perception of life.

I hope this book provides you with an explanation of Real Yoga, and the real meaning of Yoga Practice. Each and every student of Yoga is entitled to this knowledge. It is through your discipline and dedication you can transform your life to share the wisdom of the sages that came so many thousands of years ago. Through the practice of Real Yoga you will become a new person that integrates all aspect of your being with a new awareness and vision that will transcend all expectations. It will bring profound happiness to you and all the people who touch your life.

Lightning Source UK Ltd.
Milton Keynes UK
UKIC01n2006040116
265774UK00002B/10